Pharmacovigilance

*Edited by Charmy S. Kothari, Manan Shah
and Rajvi Manthan Patel*

Published in London, United Kingdom

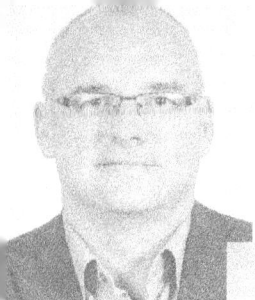
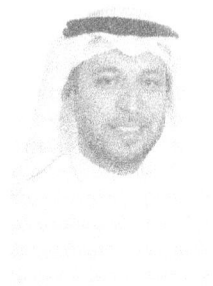
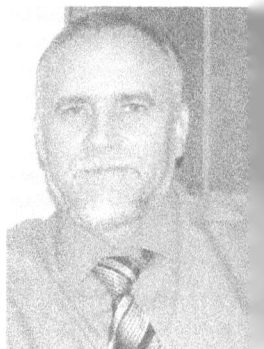
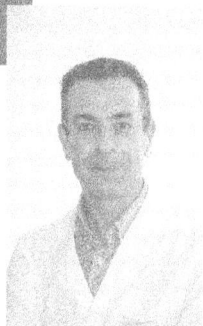
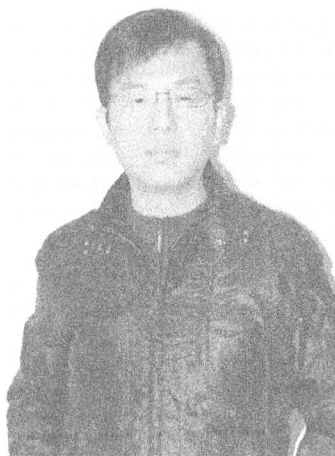
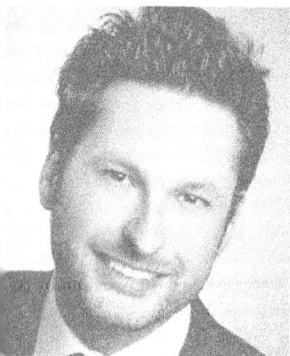
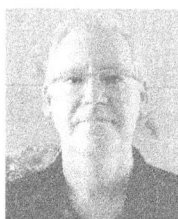

IntechOpen

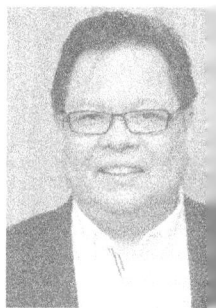
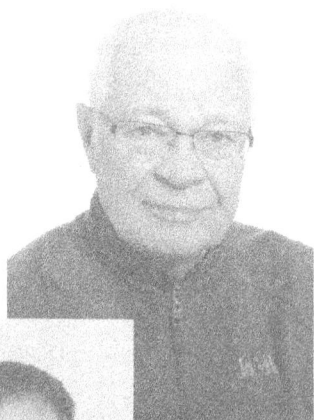
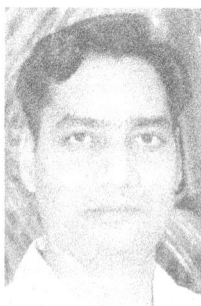
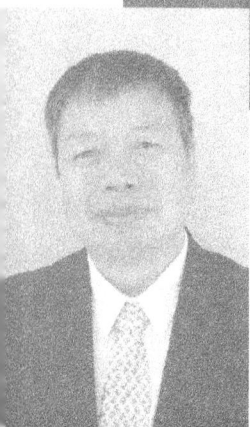
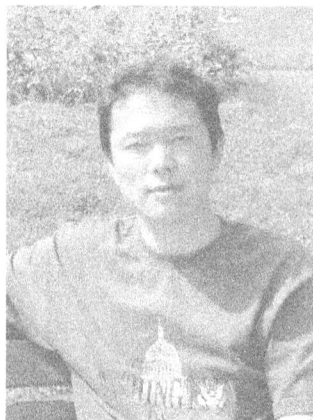
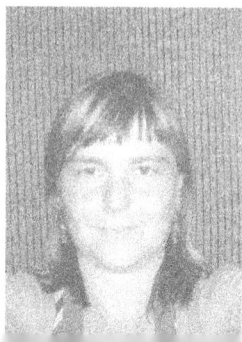

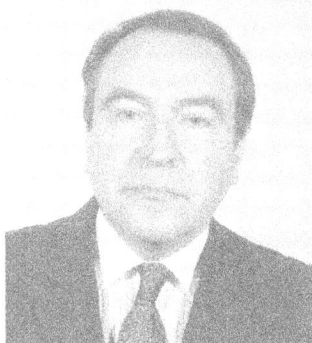

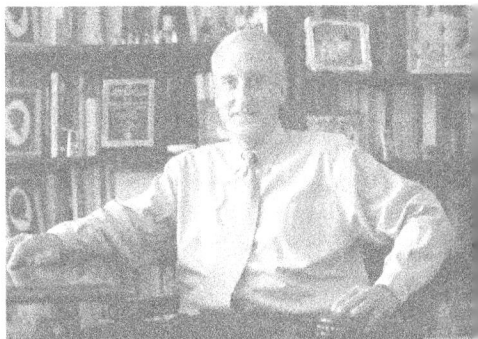

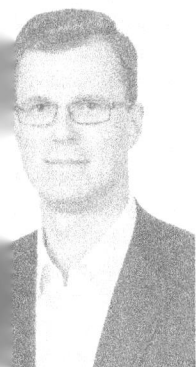

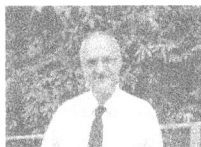

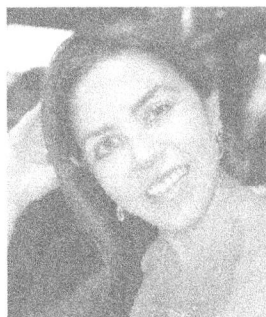

Supporting open minds since 2005

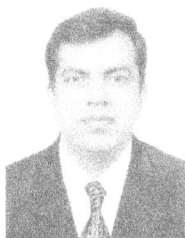

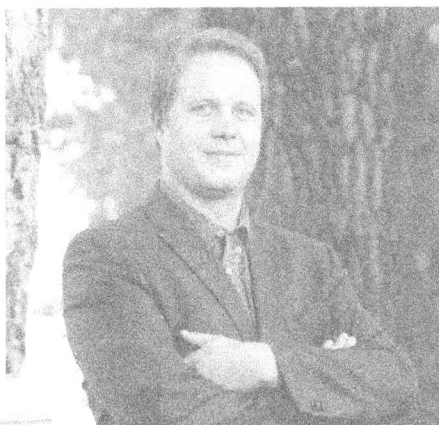

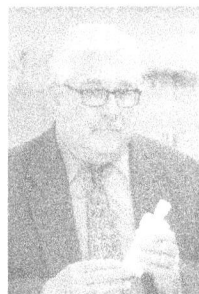

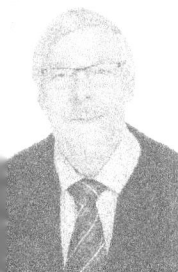

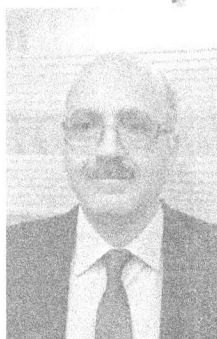

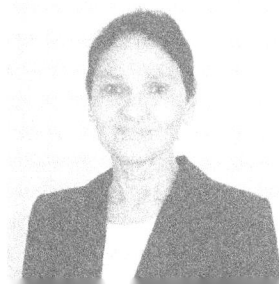

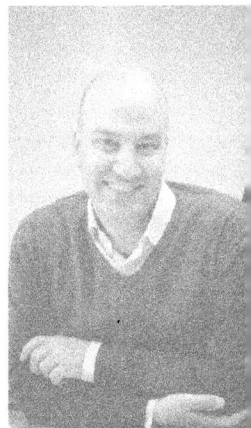

Pharmacovigilance
http://dx.doi.org/10.5772/intechopen.76269
Edited by Charmy S. Kothari, Manan Shah and Rajvi Manthan Patel

Contributors
Roxana Patricia De Las Salas-Martinez, Claudia Vásquez, Elisabetta Poluzzi, Emanuel Raschi, Fabrizio De Ponti, Ugo Moretti, Antoine Pariente, Francesco Salvo, Ippazio Cosimo Antonazzo, Pietro Fagiolino, Marta Vázquez, Cecilia Maldonado, Natalia Guevara, Manuel Ibarra, Isabel Rega, Adriana Gómez, Antonella Carozzi, Carlos Azambuja, Charmy S. Kothari, Manan Shah, Rajvi Manthan Patel

Notice
Statements and opinions expressed in the chapters are these of the individual contributors and not necessarily those of the editors or publisher. No responsibility is accepted for the accuracy of information contained in the published chapters. The publisher assumes no responsibility for any damage or injury to persons or property arising out of the use of any materials, instructions, methods or ideas contained in the book.

First published in London, United Kingdom, 2019 by IntechOpen
IntechOpen is the global imprint of INTECHOPEN LIMITED, registered in England and Wales, registration number: 11086078, The Shard, 25th floor, 32 London Bridge Street
London, SE19SG – United Kingdom
Printed in Croatia

British Library Cataloguing-in-Publication Data
A catalogue record for this book is available from the British Library

Additional hard copies can be obtained from orders@intechopen.com

Pharmacovigilance
Edited by Charmy S. Kothari, Manan Shah and Rajvi Manthan Patel
p. cm.
Print ISBN 978-1-78985-759-7
Online ISBN 978-1-78985-760-3

We are IntechOpen,
the world's leading publisher of Open Access books
Built by scientists, for scientists

4,000+
Open access books available

116,000+
International authors and editors

120M+
Downloads

Our authors are among the

151
Countries delivered to

Top 1%
most cited scientists

12.2%
Contributors from top 500 universities

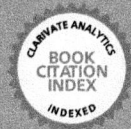

CLARIVATE ANALYTICS
BOOK
CITATION
INDEX
INDEXED

WEB OF SCIENCE™

Selection of our books indexed in the Book Citation Index
in Web of Science™ Core Collection (BKCI)

Interested in publishing with us?
Contact book.department@intechopen.com

Numbers displayed above are based on latest data collected.
For more information visit www.intechopen.com

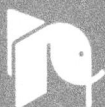

Meet the editors

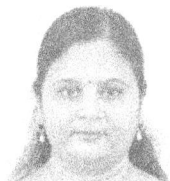

Dr. Charmy S. Kothari has more than 14 years of teaching and research experience. She has 35 research papers and review articles published in reputed Indian and International journals. She received several awards for the best oral and poster presentation and recipient of National Dr. P. D. Sethi's Award for a research paper. She is a recognized Post Graduate and Ph.D. Guide at the Institute of Pharmacy, Nirma University. To date, she has been a guide for 6 PhD and 35 M.Pharm students. She has received research grants from government funding agencies such as GUJCOST and ICMR. She received the DST-SERB International Travel Grant for attending an international conference AOAC in Canada. Her research areas of interest are stability studies, impurity profiling and isolation, identification and characterization, and the world-wide pharmacovigilance system.

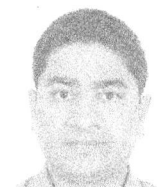

Mr. Manan Shah (B.Pharm, M.S. Forensic Pharmacy (Gold Medalist)) is currently pursuing his Ph.D. at the Institute of Pharmacy, Nirma University in the field of pharmacovigilance. Manan Shah is an active member of the International Society of Pharmacovigilance (ISOP) and has attended an international conference and workshop organized by ISOP. He has presented a paper on Pharmacovigilance in an international conference at Geneva, Switzerland. He previously worked as Assistant at the Astra Lifecare Pvt. Ltd. in the Regulatory Affairs Department. He has also worked as a Junior Research Associate at Veeda Clinical Research based at Ahmedabad. His areas of interest are Pharmacovigilance and PSUR.

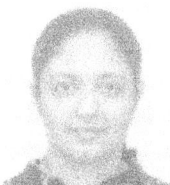

Ms. Rajvi Patel (Pharm.D) has teaching experience of more than two years and is currently engaged at the faculty at Nirma University, Institute of Pharmacy. She is currently guiding M.Pharm students in Regulatory Affairs. She also has prior experience in clinical research and the training department at Cliantha Research Limited where she was involved in training employees in various regulatory aspects. She has also worked as a registered pharmacist for two years at Basinger's Pharmacy, Illinois. She has actively participated in workshops such as medical writing and conferences such as Nipicon, 54th Indian Pharmaceutical Congress and Indian Pharmacognosy Society and ISPRA. She has presented a poster entitled "Drug abuse trends among pharmacists" during her tenure as pharmacist in USA.

Contents

Preface

The book "Pharmacovigilance" describes the pathway to understand that pharmacovigilance plays a specialized and pivotal role in ensuring ongoing safety of medicinal products. Written in plain English, the book is concise, jargon-free, facilitates an understanding of the fundamentals of pharmacovigilance, and explores regulatory aspects involved in pharmacovigilance.

Consuming a drug is equivalent to consuming a risk. It is only when the benefit associated with the drug is more than the risk, that the consumption of a drug is justified. Thus, it is the benefit versus risk ratio of the drug that decides whether a drug is to be taken or not. The next question is how to measure risks and how to measure benefits. Due to individualization of drugs to patients, it is the clinical judgment of the physician to identify what will benefit the observations related to Pharmacovigilance. The studies related to Pharmacovigilance indicate the possible risks associated with the drug.

Pharmacovigilance is an emerging area for employment in recent years. Information and in-depth knowledge of drugs is an advantage for anybody who wants to make career in this field. Hence, pharmacists are well suited to exploit the opportunity. The job potential is both local as well as global. Opportunities are enormous, one only has to make a commitment for the career.

Authors have tried to make the contents of the book more informative and inclusive; however, for an ever-changing field such as Pharmacovigilance, updates are probably a daily affair. Authors have attempted to make the content inclusive; however, comments are welcome.

Charmy Kothari
Institute of Pharmacy, Nirma University,
Ahmedabad

Manan Shah
Institute of Pharmacy, Nirma University,
India

Rajvi Manthan Patel
Institute of Pharmacy, Nirma University,
India

Basics of
Pharmacovigilance

Chapter 1

Introductory Chapter: Pharmacovigilance

Charmy S. Kothari, Manan P. Shah and Rajvi M. Patel

1. Introduction

Consuming a drug is equivalent to consume a risk. It is only when the benefit associated with the drugs are more than the risk, that the consumption of a drug is justified. Thus, it is benefit versus risk ratio of the drug which decides whether a drug is to be taken or not. The next question is how to measure risks and how to measure the benefits. Due to individualization of drugs to patients, it is the clinical judgment of the physician to identify what will benefit the patient. At the same time, risk associated with the drug can be ascertained by observations related to pharmacovigilance. The studies related to pharmacovigilance indicate what are the possible risks associated with the drug. Even drug can be associated with possible adverse reactions, intended or unintended. The only exception to this generality is the case of drug which is given in case of deficiency of specific components like vitamins or minerals. It is the study of possible adverse reactions of drugs which constitutes the essential content of Pharmacovigilance. This takes us to the definition of Pharmacovigilance.

Pharmacovigilance is the science and activities related to the detection, assessment, understanding and prevention of adverse effects or any other possible drug-related problems. [1] Spontaneous reporting of adverse events and adverse drug reactions is the commonest method utilized for generating safety data.

Major aims of pharmacovigilance are as follows:

- Early detection of hitherto unknown adverse reactions and interactions.

- Identification of risk factors and possible mechanisms underlying adverse reactions.

- Estimation of quantitative aspects of benefit/risk analysis and dissemination of information needed to improve drug prescribing and regulation.

Safety of patient is the most important when it comes about medicines. Various types of medicines are used since ancient ages and various rules and regulation were formed in modern era. If we look back in early twentieth century, the safety of patient was discussed first time when Biologics Control Act, 1902 was passed by USA [2, 3]. After that in 1962, USA promulgated a law stating that it is the manufacturer's responsibility to prove safety and efficacy of the drug before getting marketing authorization. In 1963, a committee on Safety of drugs was established in UK. In 1964, a system of "Yellow Cards" was established in UK to trace reporting safety of drugs by all users of drugs [4]. By 1964–1965, National Adverse Drugs Reaction reporting systems was initiated in countries like UK, Australia, New Zealand, Canada, West Germany and Sweden.

Year	Legislation/Act/Law/Event
1902	**Biologics Control Act** [2, 3] Passed in 1902 by USA because many deaths were reported due to diphtheria vaccines tainted with tetanus.
1906	**Pure Food and Drug Act** [5] Passed by US Congress, for preventing the manufacture, sale, or transportation of adulterated or misbranded or poisonous or deleterious foods, drugs, medicines, and liquors, and for regulating traffic therein, and for other purposes. The bill was passed after significant public pressure which resulted from a novel by the journalist Upton Sinclair which exposed unhealthy practices of the meat industry in Chicago.
1937	**Sulfanilamide Elixir** [6] used to treat streptococcal infections, which had been used without any issues in powder and tablet form. A mass poisoning of 105 patients treated with an untested medication spurred Congress to empower the US Food and Drug Administration to monitor drug safety.
1938	**Federal Food, Drug and Cosmetics Act** [7] As a result of sulfanilamide elixir incident, the Federal Food, Drugs and Cosmetics Act was passed, the statute that today remains the basis for FDA regulation.
1949	**Council for International Organizations of medical sciences (CIOMS)** [8] Established jointly by WHO and UNESCO with the objective to facilitate and promote international activities in the field of biomedical sciences, especially when the participation of several international associations and national institutions is deemed necessary.
1961	**Thalidomide tragedy** [9, 10] Thalidomide first entered the German market as an over-the-counter remedy in 1957. A German newspaper soon reported 161 babies were adversely affected by thalidomide, leading the makers of the drug—who had ignored reports of the birth defects associated with the it—to finally stop distribution within Germany. Other countries followed suit and, by March of 1962, the drug was banned in most countries where it was previously sold.
1962	**Kefauver-Harris** [11] This amendment was passed in the US Congress as a response to thalidomide tragedy. This law required evidence of drug efficacy and safety before marketing.
1964	**Yellow Card Scheme** [4] Again in the wake of thalidomide tragedy the Yellow Card Scheme (UK) was established for collecting information on suspected adverse drug reaction (ADRs) of medicine to provide an early warning of possible hazards.
1967	**WHO resolution** Resolution 20.51 laid basis for the international system of monitoring ADR.
1968	**Medicines Act** [12] Established by UK to govern the control of medicines for human and veterinary, including manufacturing and supply.
1973	**Pharmacovigilance System** [13] French Pharmacovigilance system implemented.
1982	**Benoxaprofen** [14] Was removed from the market in the UK and USA after being linked to 3500 side effects and 61 deaths. Showing that despite progress and efforts to prevent disasters, these can still occur and great care is needed to ensure patient safety.
1990	**CIOMS − 1** [15] CIOMS–1: International reporting of Adverse Drug Reactions, released.
1991	**European Rapid Alert System** Was signed into force to felicitate early exchange of information concerning possible safety hazards relating to marketing medicinal products. Reducing delay in acting on safety signals such as the case in Sulfanilamide elixir in 1937
1995	**European Medicines Agency** Established to harmonize the work of existing national medicine regulatory bodies.
2001	**EU Clinical Trial directives** [16] Issued in April 2001 and approved and implemented in May 2004.Introduced more robust measures on the safe conduct of clinical trials. Volume 9A introduced to standardize post marketing PV systems in Europe.
2009	**Black Triangle** [17] MHRA Black Triangle scheme to report all suspected adverse drug reaction to designated drugs.

Year	Legislation/Act/Law/Event
2012	**Good Pharmacovigilance Practice (GvPs)** [18]
	Release of this replaced volume 9A. It expanded and clarifies the PV responsibility of marker authorization holders.
	Regularly updated and made available for public consultation.
2014	**New Clinical Trial Regulation** [19]
	Signed into force to replace the 2001 EU-CTD. Standardized implementation across member states.

Table 1.
Roadmap of current pharmacovigilance system.

In 1962, International Center for monitoring of Adverse Drug Reaction by WHO was established in Geneva, which was later shifted to Uppsala in Sweden and this is the beginning of pharmacovigilance. From then, the WHO-supported Uppsala monitoring Centre has spearheaded many activities of pharmacovigilance all over the world (**Table 1**).

2. Current methods in pharmacovigilance

Pharmacovigilance is branch of pharmacoepidemiology but is restricted to the study, on an epidemiological scale, of drug events or adverse reactions.

Here 'events' means, recorded happenings during a period of drug monitoring in the patients notes, it may be due to the disease for which the drug is being given, some other intercurrent disease or infection, an adverse reaction to the drug being monitored or the activity of a drug being given concomitantly.

2.1 Hypothesis: generating methods

2.1.1 Spontaneous ADR reporting

Healthcare professionals are provided with forms upon which they can notify a authority of any suspected ADRs that they detect. The form is filled by healthcare professionals with direct interaction to patient after knowing the required information directly from patients. Even the consumers can directly report with the help of form.

This system remains helpful to obtain the safety information of drug throughout the lifecycle of the drug or the length of stay of the drug in the market. Spontaneous reporting has led to the identification and verification of many unexpected and serious adverse drug reaction.

2.1.2 Prescription event monitoring

This method provides the 'exposure data' showing which patients have been exposed to the drug being monitored. Strength of this method is that it provides the number of reports and the number of patients exposed both being collected over a precisely known period of time or observations.

2.1.3 Other hypothesis: generating methods

In some cases, data being collected for general public health surveillance, such as cause of death files, cancer registries and birth defect registries are used to identify patterns of events that might be associated with medication use.

2.2 Hypothesis: testing methods

2.2.1 Case-control studies

In this study, case is compared with controls susceptible to the disease but free of it. Here the exposure rate of case is compared with exposure rate in the controls. Special attention is needed in case definition so that the cases truly represent the specific outcome of interest (e.g. Stevens-Johnson syndrome and not all cases of rash).

2.2.2 Crossover design

Very useful design for the evaluation of events with onset shortly after treatment initiated. Here cases are identified not controls. A drug association is evaluated through comparing frequency of exposure at the time of the event with frequency of exposure at a different time for the same individuals. This design is less subject to bias than case–control studies because individuals serve as their own controls.

3. Causality assessment in pharmacovigilance

While reporting any adverse reaction, it is necessary to establish causal relation between the suspected drug and the observed effect. It is also possible that one of the diseases processes, interaction of the drug on disease process or even lack of effect of a drug exacerbating the disease process may be involved in the observed effect.

Causality term	Assessment criteria
Certain	Event or laboratory test abnormality, with plausible time relationship to drug intake
	• Cannot be explained by disease or other drugs
	• Response to withdrawal plausible (pharmacologically, pathologically)
	• Event definitive pharmacologically or phenomenologically (i.e. an objective and specific medical disorder or a recognized pharmacological phenomenon)
	• Rechallenge satisfactory, if necessary
Probably/ likely	• Event or laboratory test abnormality, with reasonable time relationship to drug intake
	• Unlikely to be attributed to disease or other drugs
	• Response to withdrawal clinically reasonable
	• Rechallenge not required
Possible	Event or laboratory test abnormality, with reasonable time relationship to drug intake
	• Could also be explained by disease or other drugs
	• Information on drug withdrawal may be lacking or unclear
unlikely	• Event or laboratory test abnormality, with a time to drug intake that makes a relationship improbable (but not impossible)
	• Disease or other drugs provide plausible explanations
Conditional/ unclassified	• Event or laboratory test abnormality
	• More data for proper assessment needed, or
	• Additional data under examination
Unassessable/ unclassifiable	• Report suggesting an adverse reaction
	• Cannot be judged because information is insufficient or contradictory
	• Data cannot be supplemented or verified

Table 2.
WHO-UMC system proposed by World Health Organization.

Questions	Yes	No	Do not know
Are there previous conclusion reports on this reaction?	+1	0	0
Did the adverse event appear after the suspect drug was administered?	+2	−1	0
Did the AR improve when the drug was discontinued or a specific antagonist was administered?	+1	0	0
Did the AR reappear when drug was re-administered?	+2	−1	0
Are there alternate causes [other than the drug] that could solely have caused the reaction?	−1	+2	0
Did the reaction reappear when a placebo was given?	−1	+1	0
Was the drug detected in the blood [or other fluids] in a concentration known to be toxic?	+1	0	0
Was the reaction more severe when the dose was increased or less severe when the dose was decreased?	+1	0	0
Did the patient have a similar reaction to the same or similar drugs in any previous exposure?	+1	0	0
Was the adverse event confirmed by objective evidence?	+	0	0

Scoring for Naranjo algorithm: >9 = definite ADR; 5–8 = probable ADR; 1–4 = possible ADR; 0 = doubtful ADR.

Table 3.
Naranjo ADR probability scale—items and score.

The causality assessment system proposed by the World Health Organization Collaborating Centre for International Drug Monitoring, the Uppsala Monitoring Centre (WHO–UMC) [20], and the Naranjo Probability Scale [21] are the generally accepted and most widely used methods for causality assessment in clinical practice as they offer a simple methodology (**Tables 2** and **3**).

4. Signal detection

As per World Health Organization, signal of adverse drug reaction is: "reported information on a possible causal relationship between an adverse event and a drug, the relationship being unknown or incompletely documented previously" [22].

A signal is therefore very tentative in nature; the first expression that something might be wrong with a medicinal product, or a hint given by new information which might support or explain a medicinal product–adverse reaction relationship already known [23].

Usually, more than a single report is required for signal detection (SD), depending on the seriousness of the event and the quality of the information. Once a signal is detected, one can then analyze and confirm it. In detecting signals from large ADR databases, however, one has to use a procedure that is sensitive (low false negativity) and specific (high true positivity) for the purpose [24, 25].

Different methods are being developed till today for the detection of signal. In that statistical method is very useful and very under estimated method. Such method is data mining approach, in which important and useful information are automatically and continuously extracted from large amounts of data, it is a form of exploratory data analysis and a key component of the knowledge discovery process. This approach seems particularly valuable and can be used on any large data set.

Data mining approach is divided into mainly two parts: frequentist and Bayesian methods.

Method	Advantage	Limitations	Regulatory Agencies using the method
Frequentist methods			
Proportional reporting ratio (PRR)	Easily applicable and interpretable, more sensitive compared to Bayesian method	Cannot be calculated for all drug-event combinations, low specificity	EMA (EudraVigilance), Italian Regulatory Agency
Reporting odd ratio (ROR)	Easily applicable and interpretable, more sensitive compared to Bayesian method	Odd ration cannot be calculated if denominator is zero	Lareb (Netherlands)
Bayesian methods			
Multi-item Gamma Poisson Shrinker	Always applicable, more specific as compared to frequentist methods	Relatively non transparent for people non familiar with Bayesian statistics, lower sensitivity	FDA (AERS)
Bayesian Confidence Propagation Neural Network (BCPNN)	Always applicable, more specific as compared to frequentist methods	Relatively non transparent for people non familiar with Bayesian statistics, lower sensitivity	UMC (WHO-VigiBase)

Table 4.
Data mining methods.

4.1 Frequentist method

They are particularly appealing and therefore widely used due to the fact that they are relatively easy to understand, interpret and compute as they are based on the same principles of calculation using the 2 × 2 table.

Proportional reporting ratio (PRR), Reporting odd ratio (ROR), chi-square ratio, 95% confidence interval of PRR and observed to expected ratio are calculated.

4.2 Bayesian method

Bayesian methods interpret the concept of probability as the degree to which a person believes a proposition. Bayesian inference starts with a pre-existing subjective personal assessment of the unknown parameter and the probability distribution (called prior distribution).

The signal metric or signal score in BCPNN is the information component (IC) (**Table 4**).

5. Pharmacovigilance and ICH regulations

So far, pharmacovigilance-related topics entered the ICH process in two waves. The first wave resulted in adoption of the ICH Topic ICH-E2A in 1994 with an extension to this work in the form of E2B and E2C, finalized between 1996 and 1997. The second wave started in 2002 with three further ICH topics, E2D, E2C Addendum and E2E, finalized between 2003 and 2004 (**Figure 1**).

5.1 Key points addressed in the ICH-E2A

- Definitions for AE and ADR in the pre-authorization phase [26]

- Criteria for serious AE/ADR

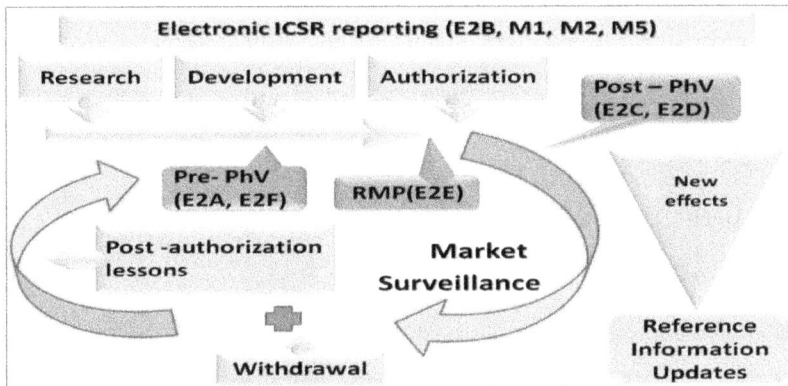

Figure 1.
Pharmacovigilance and ICH.

- Expectedness of an AE/ADR based on clinical observation and its documentation in the applicable product information

- Causality assessment as good case practice for AE/ADR cases from clinical trials

- Implied possible causality for spontaneously reported ADR cases

- Standards for expedited reporting from clinical trials

- Definition of minimum case report information for report submission to authorities

- Follow-up reporting

- Unblinding procedures for serious ADRs

- Reporting of emerging information on post-study ADRs

- Reporting requirement for active comparator

5.2 Key points addressed in the ICH-E2D

- Definitions for AE and ADR in the post-authorization phase [27]

- Criteria for serious AE/ADR in accordance with ICH-E2A

- Expectedness of an AE/ADR based on clinical observation and its documentation in the authorized product information; explanations regarding class effects

- Differentiation between sources of unsolicited and solicited reports

- Explanation on stimulated (but unsolicited) reporting

- Standards for expedited reporting in post-authorization phase

- Definition of minimum case report information for report submission to authorities with explanations

- Follow-up reporting

- Lack of efficacy reporting needs

- Guidance on ADR narratives

- Guidance on ADR case assessment

- Management of cases of exposure during pregnancy

- Explanation on reporting responsibility of marketing authorization holder despite any contractual relationship in place

5.3 Key points addressed in the ICH-E2B(M)

- Description of all data elements of ADR case reports: title and content of each data field [28]

- Technical specifications such as field length and field value for each of the data fields and the related additional technical data fields

- List of abbreviations for units

- List of units for time intervals

- List of routes of administration

5.4 Key points addressed in the ICH-E2C

- Inclusion of all product presentations in one PSUR [29]

- Concept of international birthdates of a product, determining the data lock points of PSURs

- Provision to submit a set of PSURs, each covering subsequent 6 months, to facilitate PSUR submission according to local frequency

- Description of all data sources to be covered in a PSUR

- Inclusion of worldwide information on marketing authorization status and regulatory safety-related action, ADR and exposure data

- Use of company core safety information (CCSI) as reference and concept of unlistedness of an ADR (i.e. unlisted in comparison to the CCSI versus unexpected in comparison with locally authorized product information)

- Presentation of individual case history

- Formats of ADR line listings and summary tabulations

- Presentation of exposure data

5.5 Key points addressed in the ICH-E2E

- Elements for the safety specification as summary of identified risks, risks potentially arising from populations and situations that have not yet been adequately studied and potential other risks [30]

- Format of a pharmacovigilance plan based on the safety specification

- Within the pharmacovigilance plan, the description of routine pharmaco-vigilance as minimum and inclusion of a safety action plan for specific issues/ missing information as needed

- Format of safety action plan, with the description of rationale for action and timetable for evaluation and reporting ('milestones')

- Possible synchronization of timetable with regulatory timetable for post-authorization assessment, such as PSUR assessment or marketing authoriza-tion renewal assessment

- Principles for design and conduct pharmacoepidemiological studies of non-experimental design with references to international guidelines

- Overview of methods for data collection to investigate the known or unknown risks and references

6. Pharmacovigilance in pediatric population

Pediatric population is defined as age between 0 and 18 years of age. Since many ages, pediatrician deals with limited available medicines specifically made for children. The reason behind limited availability of medicines is lack of clinical trials in this age group. Pediatricians are left with no choice other than prescribing it as "off-label" basis as these medicines have not been adequately tested and or formu-lated and authorized for use in appropriate pediatric age group. So these health care providers should be aware of risk involved in prescribing and administering such drugs to children [1].

Risk of adverse reactions increases with "off-label" use of drugs and so regula-tory authorities play an important role in reminding health care providers to report adverse drug reactions and process of pediatric pharmacovigilance [31]. Specific problems associated with pediatric population are lack of clinical trials, under or over dosage, lack of pharmacokinetics and dose-finding studies; drug induced growth and developmental disorders as well as delayed ADRs [31].

Various stakeholders that play a role in pharmacovigilance are health profession-als, parents, pharmaceutical industry, patient organizations, national healthcare systems, etc.

Different regulatory guidance's available for pediatric pharmacovigilance are but not limited to:

ICHE2E

EMEA: Guideline on conduct of pharmacovigilance for medicines used by the pediatric population.

EMEA: Guideline on conduct of pharmacovigilance for vaccines.

Points to be considered for future in pediatric pharmacovigilance are [32]:

- Pediatric population should be taken into account during all phases of pharmacovigilance cycle

- Encourage ADR reporting

- Expanding definition of ADR to include off-label, misuse, error.

- Risk management plans

- Signal detecting systems

- Additional monitoring system

7. The future

The drugs can viewed, in general terms, like any other commodity. Patients will be able to choose what is best for them on the basis of information they are given. Drugs with relatively less benefit or more risk will find an appropriate market level. We believe this involves the public understanding more about benefit and risk, more suitable information coming from regulators and industry regarding benefit and risk of drugs, health professionals being able to interpret information for singular situations and the law and media playing a more constructive role in the whole process. The situation is undoubtedly more complicated than this, and the issues of communications in a crisis involving safety issues with a drug not only affect the situation but have a more general impact. These high profiles issues deserve special attention as does the impact of new communications media and sources.

Pharmacovigilance benefits everybody. The patients are protected from unsafe drugs, doctors and pharmaceutical industry keep their reputations intact and drug regulators receive pertinent data that helps them to take regulatory decisions.

It is expected that with the involvement of all related stakeholders, Pharmacovigilance program will help in reducing the cost of damages caused by drugs to minimal level. It will also try to prevent drug-related damages if appropriate care is taken by physicians on the basis of feedback from the pharmacovigilance program.

Author details

Charmy S. Kothari*, Manan P. Shah and Rajvi M. Patel
Institute of Pharmacy, Nirma University, Ahmedabad, India

*Address all correspondence to: charmyshah@gmail.com;
charmy.kothari@nirmauni.ac.in

IntechOpen

References

[1] WHO. Pharmacovigilance. Available from: http://www.who.int/medicines/areas/quality_safety/safety_efficacy/pharmvigi/en/ [Accessed: September 11, 2018]

[2] A Short History of the National Institutes of Health. Available from: https://history.nih.gov/exhibits/history/docs/page_03.html [Accessed: September 11, 2018]

[3] Bren L. The road to the biotech revolution: Highlights of 100 years of biologics regulation. FDA Consum. **40**:50-57

[4] Yellow Card Scheme—MHRA. Available from: https://yellowcard.mhra.gov.uk/the-yellow-card-scheme/ [Accessed: September 11, 2018]

[5] Food and Drug Act of 1906. Encyclopedia.com. Available from: https://www.encyclopedia.com/history/united-states-and-canada/us-history/food-and-drug-act-1906 [Accessed: September 11, 2018]

[6] Akst J. The Elixir Tragedy, 1937 | The Scientist Magazine®. https://www.the-scientist.com/foundations/the-elixir-tragedy-1937-39231, [Accessed December 13, 2018]

[7] FDA Basics—How did the Federal Food, Drug, and Cosmetic Act Come About? Available from: https://www.fda.gov/aboutfda/transparency/basics/ucm214416.htm [Accessed: September 11, 2018]

[8] Our History—CIOMS. Available from: https://cioms.ch/history/ [Accessed: September 11, 2018]

[9] Kim JH, Scialli AR. Thalidomide: The tragedy of birth defects and the effective treatment of disease. Toxicological Sciences. 2011;**122**:1-6

[10] Thalidomide Embryopathy Report of a meeting of experts World Health Organization (WHO), Geneva, 2014. p. 1-26

[11] Greene JA, Podolsky SH. Reform, regulation, and pharmaceuticals—The Kefauver-Harris amendments at 50. The New England Journal of Medicine. 2012;**367**:1481-1483

[12] Medicines Act 1968, United Kingdom Legislative Body, London. 1968

[13] Welsch M, Alt M, Richard MH, Imbs JL. The French pharmacovigilance system: Structure and missions. Presse Médicale. 2000;**29**:102-106

[14] Lowe D. When Drug Launches Go Bad | In the Pipeline. https://blogs.sciencemag.org/pipeline/archives/2012/11/29/when_drug_launches_go_bad, (Accessed December 13, 2018)

[15] Pharmacovigilance—CIOMS. Available from: https://cioms.ch/pharmacovigilance/becoming-the-cioms-member-2/ [Accessed: September 11, 2018]

[16] Directive 2001/20/EC of the European Parliament and of the Council of 4 April 2001 on the Approximation of the Laws, Regulations and Administrative Provisions of the Member States Relating to the Implementation of Good Clinical Practice in the Conduct of Clinical Trials on Medicinal Products for Human Use. Available from: https://www.eortc.be/services/doc/clinical-eu-directive-04-april-01.pdf [Accessed: September 11, 2018]

[17] Black Triangle Scheme-new medicines and vaccines subject to EU-wide additional monitoring, London. 2009

[18] Guideline on good pharmacovigilance practices (GVP) Module I – Pharmacovigilance systems and their quality systems, European Medicines Agency, London. 2012

[19] European Medicines Agency. Clinical Trials—Clinical Trial Regulation. Available from: http://www.ema.europa.eu/ema/index.jsp?curl=pages/regulation/general/general_content_000629.jsp [Accessed: September 11, 2018]

[20] World Health Organization. The use of the WHO-UMC system for standardized case causality assessment. Uppsala: The Uppsala Monitoring Centre. 2005:2-7

[21] Naranjo CA, Busto U, Sellers EM, Sandor P, Ruiz I, Roberts EA, et al. A method for estimating the probability of adverse drug reactions. Clinical Pharmacology and Therapeutics. 1981;**30**:239-245

[22] UMC. Signal Detection. Available from: https://www.who-umc.org/research-scientific-development/signal-detection/ [Accessed: September 13, 2018]

[23] Mann RD, Andrews EB. PHARMACOVIGILANCE Second Edition, John Wiley and Sons, Ltd, West Sussex, Second., 2007

[24] Chakraborty BS. Pharmacovigilance: A data mining approach to signal detection. Indian Journal of Pharmacology. 2015;**47**:241-242

[25] Wilson AM, Thabane L, Holbrook A. Application of data mining techniques in pharmacovigilance. British Journal of Clinical Pharmacology. 2004;**57**:127-134

[26] International Conference on Harmonisation Working Group. ICH harmonised tripartite guideline: Clinical Safety Data Management: Definations and standards for expedited reporting (E2A). International Conference on Harmonisation of Technical Requirements for Registration of Pharmaceuticals for Human Use. Oct 1994

[27] International Conference on Harmonisation Working Group. ICH harmonised tripartite guideline: Post Approval safety data management: Definations and standards for expedited reporting (E2D). International Conference on Harmonisation of Technical Requirements for Registration of Pharmaceuticals for Human Use. Nov 2003

[28] International Conference on Harmonisation Working Group. ICH harmonised tripartite guideline: Implementation working group electronic transmission of individual case safety reports (ICSRs) questions and answers, E2B(R3). International Conference on Harmonisation of Technical Requirements for Registration of Pharmaceuticals for Human Use. 2004

[29] International Conference on Harmonisation Working Group. ICH harmonised tripartite guideline: Periodic benefit-risk evaluation report (PBRER). International Conference on Harmonisation of Technical Requirements for Registration of Pharmaceuticals for Human Use. Dec 2012

[30] International Conference on Harmonisation Working Group. ICH harmonised tripartite guideline: Pharmacovigilance Planning (E2E). International Conference on Harmonisation of Technical Requirements for Registration of Pharmaceuticals for Human Use. Nov 2004

[31] Cristiana Scasserra EN. Pharmacovigilance in Pediatric Age: The

Role of Family Pediatricians-Medicines
for Children Research Network
(FP-MCRN), J. Pharmacovigil.
2015;**03**:1-6

[32] Raine JM. An agency of the
European Union Pharmacovigilance
in Paediatric Population The PRAC's
perspective, London. 2014

Evolving Roles of Spontaneous Reporting Systems to Assess and Monitor Drug Safety

Emanuel Raschi, Ugo Moretti, Francesco Salvo,

Antoine Pariente, Ippazio Cosimo Antonazzo,

Fabrizio De Ponti and Elisabetta Poluzzi

Abstract

This chapter aims to describe current and emerging roles of spontaneous reporting systems (SRSs) for assessing and monitoring drug safety. Moreover, it offers a perspective on the near future, which entails the so-called era of Big Data, keeping in mind both regulator and researcher viewpoints. After a panorama on key data sources and analyses of post-marketing data of adverse drug reactions, a critical appraisal of methodological issues and debated future applications of SRSs will be presented, including the exploitation and challenges in evidence integration (i.e., merging and combining heterogeneous sources of data into a unique indicator of risk) and patient's reporting via social media. Finally, a call for a responsible use of these studies is offered, with a proposal on a set of minimum requirements to assess the quality of disproportionality analysis in terms of study conception, performing and reporting.

Keywords: pharmacovigilance, signal, spontaneous reporting system, disproportionality analysis

1. Introduction

Prescription of a medication is based on a balance between expected benefits, already investigated before marketing authorization, and possible risks (i.e., adverse effects), which become fully apparent only as time goes by after marketing authorization. Premarketing development, in fact, provides evidence on efficacy of drugs in ideal clinical setting of use (i.e., clinical trials); only the most frequent side effects are recognized in this step. The use of drugs in the real-world circumstances will show the actual risk-benefit profile.

The World Health Organization (WHO) previously defined **pharmacovigilance (PhV)** as "the science and activities relating to the detection, assessment, understanding and prevention of adverse effects or any other possible drug-related problems" [1], a definition that, in the recent past, was regarded as being synonymous with post-marketing surveillance for adverse drug reactions (ADRs).

After the adoption in 2012 of the new pharmacovigilance legislation (**Regulation (EU) No 1235/2010 and Directive 2010/84/EU**) [2, 3] approved by the European Parliament and European Council in December 2010, PhV embraces the whole risk-benefit assessment, thus dealing with multiple types of evidence emerging along the life cycle of drugs for continuous reassessment of the place in therapy of each medicine, both in clinical and in regulatory terms.

Many sources of data and relevant methods of analysis are used in PhV: from disproportionality analyses (DAs) in spontaneous reporting systems (SRSs) to analytical studies (cohort or case-control designs). These traditional approaches are now integrated by innovative strategies (e.g., social media mining and case-population studies) in the **fourth-generation PhV** [4].

In this chapter, current and emerging roles of DAs in SRSs will be critically discussed, keeping in mind both regulator and researcher viewpoints. A panorama on key data sources (and their proper selection) will be described, followed by a critical appraisal of methodological issues and debated future applications, including exploitation and challenges in evidence integration (i.e., merging and combining heterogeneous sources of data into a unique indicator of risk) and patient's reporting *via* social media. All these issues are based on key publications of the authors and on the latest advances published in the literature (MEDLINE, as of May 1, 2018). Finally, a call for a responsible use of these studies is offered, with a proposal (authors' personal ideas) on a set of minimum requirements to assess the quality of DAs in terms of study conception, performing and reporting.

2. Post-marketing data sources

Not only notification of suspected adverse drug events is mandatory for health professionals, but also other subjects can report events to the relevant regulatory authorities. According to ICH-E2 guidelines (International Conference on Harmonization, http://www.ich.org/products/guidelines/efficacy/article/efficacy-guidelines.html), each National Drug Agency maintains its specific SRS to collect all notifications and routinely use data-mining algorithms (DMAs) to process data, with the aim of identifying possible signals of unknown drug-effect associations. These DMAs identify drug-reaction pairs occurring with a significant disproportion in comparison with all other pairs, through the method of *case-non case approach*. Reactions are usually recorded according to the "MedDRA" classification (medical dictionary for regulatory activities), which allows to select cases at different hierarchical levels (from SOC—system organ class to PT—preferred term; https://www.meddra.org/).

Clinical pharmacology knowledge is requested to design and interpret results from DMAs and to decide if further examination is needed (either within the same source of data or by other types of data) or specific bias affects the validity of the findings. Other healthcare data sources are available for PhV to corroborate results of SRS data mining, despite developed for other reasons. As a general classification, they can be pooled into two main groups: electronic medical records (EMRs) and claim databases.

Electronic medical records (EMRs) aim to assist physicians in daily clinical practice (including appropriate prescription) by collecting sociodemographic and clinical information (diagnoses, risk factors, treatments, and outcomes). Primary care is the most frequent setting to develop these kinds of databases such as Clinical Practice Research Datalink (CPRD; formerly General Practice Research Database—GPRD, in UK); Health Search (by the Italian College of General Practitioners); The Health Improvement Network (THIN), in UK; and Interdisciplinary Processing of Clinical Information (IPCI), in the Netherlands. The high quantity of data makes them valuable sources to address clinical pharmacology questions, including new effects of drugs (especially on primary endpoints, to confirm premarketing evidence) and assessment of appropriate drug use (closer to the main purpose of the registries).

Claim databases were mainly created for administrative purposes, and together with hospital databases provide valuable sources to address PhV questions: data provided (e.g., diagnoses of hospital admissions, reimbursed prescriptions of drugs and diagnostic procedures in ambulatory care) are generally used for reimbursement and other economic issues, and, as a secondary aim, they represent an important source of information for epidemiological questions (taking into account that nonreimbursed intervention is usually not recorded, information on lifestyle and actual exposure to medicines is lacking.

3. Main spontaneous reporting systems

Each National Drug Agency collects its own reports in a dedicated spontaneous reporting database, and some international SRSs gather reports originating both by systematic flows from national databases and by direct submission of the reporter. Each source has specific characteristics and limitations to be considered when planning a drug safety analysis (e.g., completeness of data and options for database interrogation); however, collecting information from all these accessible sources is the mainstay in PhV.

Table 1 shows an overview of main international PhV databases, which cover a very large population and heterogeneous patterns of drug use and ADR reporting attitudes. Public access to SRSs is becoming a standard, as addressed in Section 8.2.

4. The appropriate choice of data source according to the research question

The identification of the most appropriate source of data is a key step to properly address the research question, considering strength and limitations of the different approaches (**Table 2**). For instance, SRSs represent the best source of data to investigate the so-called designated medical events (DMEs), usually rare with strong drug-attributable component (e.g., Torsades de Pointes and Stevens-Johnson Syndrome) [5, 6]. Conversely, possible role of drugs in events with high background incidence (e.g., myocardial infarction) can be better investigated by healthcare databases (EMRs and claim databases) [7, 8]. No matter of the type of ADR, a typical time sequence to detect safety profile of drugs considers data mining of SRSs as the first step of the analysis, followed by investigation through healthcare databases to confirm or refuse statistically significant associations.

From data cleaning (a mere data managing step, see later) to statistical analyses, all steps of data management are considered tasks to address questions on ADRs. Usually, each source of data requires specific data-mining approaches (e.g., disproportion calculation for SRSs and multiple regression analysis for EMRs), but emergent strategies to better exploit the more accessible sources are now appearing in the literature (e.g., self-controlled time series and prescription sequence symmetry analysis—PSSA) [9]. In fact, data mining could virtually provide as many associations as possible between drug and effect, but without consensus among experts on the methodological steps and confirmation of pathophysiological pathways, the association can easily conduct to interpret errors.

	FAERS	WHO—VigiBase	EudraVigilance	Australian Database of Adverse Event Notifications (DAEN)	Canada Vigilance Adverse Reaction Online Database	Japanese Adverse Drug Event Report database (JADER)
Website	http://www.fda.gov/Drugs/GuidanceComplianceRegulatoryInformation/Surveillance/AdverseDrugEffects/default.htm	http://www.vigiaccess.org	http://www.adrreports.eu	https://www.tga.gov.au/database-adverse-event-notifications-daen	https://www.canada.ca/en/health-canada/services/drugs-health-products/medeffect-canada/adverse-reaction-database.html	http://www.pmda.go.jp/
Access	Full data access (download) since 2004[a]	Web-based interface (VigiLize™, VigiFlow™, VigiMine, applications for full data access[c])	Web-based interface (different access policies for full data access[d])		Full data access (download)	Full data access (download)
Timeframe	1969–present	1968–present	2001–present	1971–present	1965–present	2004–present
Products covered	All drugs and biologics[b]	All drugs and biologics, including vaccines	All drugs and biologics authorized in the European Union	All medicines, including vaccines, used in Australia[e]	All drugs, biologics, vaccines, and natural health products licensed in Canada[f]	All drugs and biologics, including vaccines used in Japan

	FAERS	WHO—VigiBase	EudraVigilance	Australian Database of Adverse Event Notifications (DAEN)	Canada Vigilance Adverse Reaction Online Database	Japanese Adverse Drug Event Report database (JADER)
Source of reports	Healthcare professionals, drug companies, patients/consumers	National and regional pharmacovigilance centers (which may receive reports from patients, healthcare professionals, or drug companies)	National competent authorities and marketing authorization holders (currently, no direct reporting from patients and healthcare professionals)	Healthcare professionals, consumers, and market authorization holders	Healthcare professionals, consumers, and market authorization holders	Healthcare professionals, consumers, and market authorization holders
Current number of reports available	>12 million (as of April 2015), more than 1,000,000 per year (2012–2014)	>10 million (as of 2016)	>1 million received in 2013	Unknown (no public statistics provided)	Unknown (no public statistics provided)	~500,000 (as of 2017)
Origin of submitted reports	USA and serious/unexpected reports from EU, Japan, and other extra-US countries	Worldwide (107 official members and 33 associate members), but majority from EU and the US	EU	Australia	Canada	Japan

	FAERS	WHO—VigiBase	EudraVigilance	Australian Database of Adverse Event Notifications (DAEN)	Canada Vigilance Adverse Reaction Online Database	Japanese Adverse Drug Event Report database (JADER)
Coding system for event	MedDRA	MedDRA	MedDRA	MedDRA	MedDRA	MedDRA
Search strategy through "free text" in the narratives	No (a Freedom of Information Act can be requested to the FDA)	No	No	No	No	No

Modified and updated from [32, 113]. ADR: adverse drug reaction; MedDRA: Medical Dictionary for Regulatory Activities.

[a]*Different web-based tools are provided; see Böhm et al. [14]. Recently, the FDA has launched the FAERS Public Dashboard, a highly interactive web-based tool that allows to query FAERS data in a user-friendly fashion (https://fis.fda.gov/sense/app/777e9f4d-0cf8-448e-8068-f564-31baa25/sheet/7a4fa261-d58b-4203-a8aa-6d3021737452/state/analysis).*

[b]*Devices, vaccines, and other products are not included, as they are specifically recorded in ad hoc databases: MAUDE—Manufacturer and User Facility Device Experience (ttps://www.accessdata.fda.gov/scripts/cdrh/cfdocs/cfMAUDE/search.CFM), VAERS—Vaccines Adverse Event Reporting System (https://vaers.hhs.gov/data/datasets.html), and CAERS—Center for Food Safety and Applied Nutrition Adverse Event Reporting System (https://www.fda.gov/food/complianceenforcement/ucm494015.htm).*

[c]*Freely available for all members in the WHO Program for International Drug Monitoring.*

[d]*Specific access policies are described depending on stakeholder groups. For details, see the following link: http://www.ema.europa.eu/ema/index.jsp?curl=pages/news_and_events/news/2011/07/news_detail_001299.jsp&murl=menus/news_and_events.jsp&mid=WC0b01ac05800-4d5c1. On November 22, 2017, a new and improved version of EudraVigilance was launched. The new system has enhanced features for the reporting and analysis of suspected adverse reactions to support a better safety monitoring of medicines and a more efficient reporting process for stakeholders.*

[e]*Medical devices are not included, as they are specifically recorded in the ad hoc Database of Adverse Event Notifications—medical devices (http://apps.tga.gov.au/prod/DEVICES/daen-entry.aspx).*

[f]*Data on human blood and blood components have only been included since September 1, 2015; data on vaccines used for immunization have only been included since January 1, 2011; the majority of vaccine reports are submitted to the Canadian Adverse Events Following Immunization Surveillance System (CAEFISS).*

Table 1.
Overview of major international spontaneous reporting systems that can be searched via online systems.

	Strengths	Weaknesses
Disproportionality approach	It can be conducted rapidly, and it is easy to implement. It can be conducted on spontaneous reporting systems and healthcare databases. Good performance (accuracy in discriminating false from true positives) when major confounders and biases are accounted for. Highly suitable for rare events with high drug-attributable risk (e.g., TdP and DILI).	Does not provide risk estimates. Loss of information due to aggregated data. Unable to handle numerous confounders. Sensitive to protopathic and indication biases. Less suitable for events with high background incidence (e.g., myocardial infarction).
Traditional pharmacoepidemiological designs	It provides risk estimates (cohort and case-control design). It allows controlling for confounders if matching and nesting are performed (case-control design). Robust to confounders that are stable over time (case crossover, self-controlled cohort, and self-controlled case series). Highly suitable for events with high background incidence (e.g., myocardial infarction).	It needs very large dataset to have enough power to detect signals in case of rare events (cohort and case-control design). Less suitable for rare events with high drug-attributable risk (e.g., TdP and DILI).
Prescription sequence symmetry analysis (PSSA)	Rapid and easy to be performed (it only requires patient identifier, medication code, and medication dispensed date). Graphical output can be generated to help data visualization and interpretation. Highly specific and moderate sensitivity. It can control for time-constant confounders.	It does not provide risk estimates (it complements disproportionality approach). Prescribing trends are affected by external factors (adjustment is required). Inappropriate identification of new use (exclusion/censoring of switchers is required). Time-variant confounders. Sensitive to inverse causality, protopathic, and indication biases.
Systematic review with meta-analysis	It can provide risk estimates (especially if RCT is the primary source). It does not require additional data collection. It can be conducted rapidly. It can highlight gaps in research.	Validity depends on the scientific rigor of the methods, quality, and type of primary source (RCT or observational studies). Meta-analysis of nonrandomized studies (observational) is currently not standardized.

Modified from [9]. DILI: drug-induced liver injury; RCT: randomized controlled trial; TdP: torsade de pointes.

Table 2.
Overview of study designs to assess safety of medicines.

5. Current applications of disproportionality analyses and case-by-case assessment

5.1 The regulator's view

Traditionally, regulatory decision-making has relied on detection of safety signals through spontaneous reports. Today, things are changing for several reasons, including increased awareness of prescribers on the importance of PhV and the emerging role of different health professionals and patients.

A modern model involves signal detection, signal validation (i.e., signal should represent a novel causal relationship between a drug and an event), signal prioritization (evaluation of clinical impact of the safety issue), and some other steps to drive the decision-making, also on the basis of data on how drugs are used in a population and how their utilization can be influenced. Drug consumption is also now frequently analyzed by regulators to evaluate the actual impact of risk minimization strategies in a specific settings, such as the risk of progressive multifocal leukoencephalopathy with multiple sclerosis therapies [10].

Regulatory agencies routinely perform analyses of SRSs to detect disproportionality signals, especially for new drugs. Although the Food and Drug Administration (FDA) and the European Medicine Agency (EMA) have different frameworks, they are promoting rigorous scientific information exchange for optimal post-approval drug safety monitoring [11]. Both agencies publicly posted the list of signals emerging from internal analyses, with the aim to promote transparency and stimulate research while avoiding alarm. Usually, many of these signals remain (fortunately) unnoticed by clinicians, and only a minority of them result in measures affecting clinical practice, such as ketoacidosis with sodium-glucose cotransporter-2 inhibitors, which in turn prompted the FDA to revise relevant labels.

Also for old drugs, the importance of spontaneous reports should not be overlooked, especially because the amount of time of a drug on the market (drug age) is correlated with the number of signals detected [12]. The recent case of tiocolchicoside, restricted in recommended dose and treatment duration by the EMA, is noteworthy: after withdrawal of tetrazepam, the use of alternatives (including tiocolchicoside) and relevant spontaneous reporting increased, which made evident specific safety concerns [13].

In the past, regulatory actions on a given safety issue did not support clinical practice. The case of haloperidol and the risk of torsade de pointes (TdP) is a typical example: an ECG before administration was indeed recommended in some circumstances before administering the medicine. However, it was not duly taken into account that a psychotic crisis does not usually allow appropriate ECG measurement, and this results in the inability to use injectable haloperidol in the emergency setting. The clinical consequence was a loss of this therapeutic option and its substitution with alternatives, which are not necessarily better.

5.2 The researcher's view

Disproportionality analyses (DAs) are attracting considerable interest in the medical literature for several reasons:

1. there is increasing availability of publicly accessible SRSs and open-access tools to independently analyze international databases [14]; the various web-based resources mainly differ in terms of data transparency, possibility to customize searches and analyses (e.g., correction for confounders);

2. DAs are inexpensive and relatively quick and easy to perform, at least by frequentist methods such as reporting odds ratio (ROR) and proportional

reporting ratio (PRR); these methods can be applied systematically to analyze a given pharmacological class or specific DMEs such as TdP [15];

3. they are likely to be published in a high ranking journal, especially when sophisticated analyses are presented, claiming to correct for multiple confounders [16], and a strong signal emerges. This aspect raises ethical issues: on one hand, the researcher may be more prone toward an alarming interpretation of the findings to increase the impact of the publication. On the other hand, when broadly looking at the published literature in the past 5 years, only a minority of industry-sponsored studies provided "negative findings," that is, the lack of statistically significant DAs [17, 18].

This "uncontrolled" scenario has generated what someone coined "apophenia," that is, the perception of meaningful patterns and causal connections among random data [19], or the so-called pharmacovigilance syndrome, that is, the incorrect use of spontaneous adverse event reports to infer that a drug causes an adverse reaction, what the incidence or prevalence of such events may be, and whether one drug has lower or higher risk than another [20]. This in turn increases the complexity in the risk-benefit assessment [21] and may generate false alarm among clinicians [22].

It must be emphasized that statistical techniques, usually referred to as quantitative analyses [23], cannot be used as a standalone approach to assess a drug-related risk because no risk quantification can be offered: they should be viewed in conjunction with a qualitative analysis of individual reports, whenever feasible, and other pieces of evidence (e.g., observational studies). In other words, they cannot replace a proper clinical judgment in the individual patient.

In the recent past, a debate arose on the proper use of DAs and the benefit of their publication [24, 25]. However, no actions have been taken so far. The key applications of DAs are summarized as follows:

A. **Signal detection** (including specific events or the overall safety profile). This is the main goal of DAs, especially for medicines with unpredictable pharmacokinetics-pharmacodynamics such as biologicals [26], or recently marketed drugs with still undefined safety profile. This is also justified for rare adverse events that may escape detection in premarketing clinical trials (e.g., TdP, liver injury) or in case an imbalance (not reaching statistical significance) emerged from clinical data, as happened for pioglitazone and bladder cancer [27]. The choice of comparator group is pivotal in signal detection, especially in terms of clinical implications. For instance, a novel antidiabetic drug should be compared with other antidiabetic drugs through the so-called analysis by therapeutic area (i.e., comparing the reporting of a given drug with other agents belonging to the same therapeutic class), in order to identify patients that are likely to share the common risk factors, mitigate the confounding by indication bias, and investigate the potential intraclass variations of risk [28–32]. As a matter of fact, a suspected risk for a drug can be interpreted by a clinical point of view only if compared to the same risk of therapeutic alternatives, especially for severe disorders (e.g., diabetes) because patient cannot be left without treatment.

B. **Test/verify/confirm a pharmacological hypothesis.** This can be illustrated by a number of examples in the recent past, including the relationship between hERG blockade and occurrence of TdP in humans [33]; the risk of diabetes by antipsychotics, which was more frequently associated with agents blocking simultaneously histamine H1 and serotonin 5-HT2C receptors [34]; the association between different receptor occupancy and antipsychotic-induced movement disorders [35], and the link between dopamine receptor agonist drugs and specific impulse control disorders [36].

C. **Address/verify methodological issues.** This aspect is receiving an increasing attention because it may strongly impact on final results. Before planning the analysis, it is important to verify all potential biases affecting the drug(s) or event(s) under investigation and prespecify strategies to handle with these confounders (see Section 7) [37–43].

D. **Investigate the likelihood of drug-drug interactions.** A few pilot initiatives proposed theoretical strategies as well as relevant automated methods to detect signals resulting from drug-drug interactions (DDIs) in PhV databases [44–48]. Various approaches can be used to highlight adverse drug interactions: (a) reported suspicion of interactions as noted by the reporter in a case narrative, (b) assignment of the two drugs as interacting (c) drug-drug interaction reported as adverse event, and (d) increased co-reporting for the drug pair when disproportionality is applied [49]. There is also interest in using SRSs to investigate whether a given drug-drug combination moderates the frequency of an adverse event [50, 51].

A recent systematic review highlighted that only a minority of studies aimed at confirming or supporting previous regulatory decisions on a given safety aspect [52], thus strengthening the aforementioned concept that DAs do not usually support, on their own, regulatory actions but must be integrated with other data sources.

Apart from DAs, the value of case-by-case assessment should not be disregarded. In fact, the individual evaluation of reports performed by pharmacovigilance experts with medical background has multiple aims: (a) it may *per se* be used for signal detection of rare ADRs, such as in the case of DMEs by detecting potential drug-event combinations even earlier than DAs [53] and (b) it may confirm or refuse disproportionality signals, by strengthening/reducing causality assessment or by identifying duplicates by automated strategy (through the use of narratives). The key challenging aspect of case-by-case analysis is represented by causality assessment, that is, the process of differential diagnoses to prove actual causal relationship: exclusion of alternative causes, biological and temporal plausibility, evidence of dechallenge and rechallenge (usually unintentional) should be verified. The complexity of causality assessment stems from the fact that it needs to be viewed from the context of the patient treated rather than the drug product [54]. Although several approaches are available to assess causality, no single method is universally accepted and there is no *gold standard* [55]. The choice of the most suitable approach may also depend on the event under investigation; for instance, ALDEN is a specific algorithmic score validated for assessment of drug causality in Stevens-Johnson syndrome/toxic epidermal necrolysis [56], whereas Roussel Uclaf Causality Assessment Method (RUCAM) was implemented for drug-induced liver injury [57].

As a conclusive remark, it should be recognized that most researchers are from academia, and in fact, their additional role is university teaching. In the last few years, experts of medical teaching have strengthened the importance of PhV in the core curriculum of undergraduate students of healthcare courses (i.e., medicine, pharmacy, dentistry, nursing, etc.). WHO and the most active national PhV centers are committed to better define knowledge, skills, and attitudes that students should acquire in order to have an active role in pharmacovigilance [58].

6. Potential future applications: evidence integration and risk estimates

Integration of heterogeneous data (literature including mass media, clinical trials, observational studies, spontaneous reporting data analysis, case reports, and preclinical data) is currently in the research domain at the preliminary level, with the degree of confidence and reliance on a given source as key unresolved issues. An attempt to achieve a risk score on the pro-arrhythmic potential of drugs was undertaken within the ARITMO project [59], where a Dempster-Shafer model was used to combine evidence from heterogeneous and independent sources using expert judgment [60]. The only published experience on data integration in pharmacovigilance comes from the (useful) interplay between SRSs and healthcare databases to increase the accuracy of signal detection [61, 62].

In the following section, the issue of evidence integration for research purposes will be addressed in the context of systematic reviews, which are increasingly being used as they can make researchers and readers aware about what is known, how it is known, how evidence varies across studies, and thus about what is not already known [63].

Issues of data quality and inherent limitations cause remarkable impact in spontaneous reporting studies in which more sources of variability (e.g., missing data) and biases affecting the results could be identified (competition or notoriety bias). Nevertheless, so far, no specific tools or techniques have been developed to select, compare, or pool together data from DAs. This could be due to a relative paucity of this kind of analysis in the medical literature.

Disproportionality is used to detect "signals of disproportionate reporting" (SDRs) that, once detected, are usually investigated through other, and more precisely, study designs. It is thus rare to have additional DAs regarding the same outcome related to the same drug or drug class and that used a comparable tool for signal detection (frequentist vs. Bayesian approaches). Nevertheless, at least theoretically, techniques and statistical basis used to perform meta-analysis could also be used to analyze results from disproportionality, at least to evaluate consistency of signal across different databases. A consistent signal found in two databases could be probably prioritized in comparison with inconsistent ones. Notably, raw data cannot be pooled because of the existence of an unquantified degree of redundancy (i.e., duplicates across databases), but results can be combined to reach a single "pharmacovigilance score" [59].

It is well known that results of DA cannot be considered as measures of risk: the number of cases in a spontaneous reporting database does correspond to neither the number of cases that happened under the drug nor to that of cases induced by the drug, and the number of exposed people is not measured. From this point of view, including results of disproportionality in a meta-analysis could be considered inappropriate, although identification of heterogeneity in reporting may be of interest [64]. In the absence of any clear guideline, disproportionality studies could be searched and included in (qualitative) systematic reviews, but their results must be kept separated from pooled risk estimates of (quantitative) meta-analyses [65]. A recent experience by a French team on safety of drugs acting on the nitric oxide pathway in pulmonary hypertension considers together results from a DA of VigiBase and from a meta-analysis of clinical trials and concludes that the safety profiles of riociguat and phosphodiesterase inhibitors were different, thus providing a rationale for safe prescribing [66]. This approach, as the integration of spontaneous reporting analysis in meta or teleoanalysis [67], is still a research question.

Preliminary findings raise the hypothesis that, provided that all technical and clinical aspects are addressed, the performance of DAs is remarkable [7] and may approach the relative risks of analytical studies, thus providing an initial indication of the likely clinical importance of an adverse event [68].

7. Methodological aspects

7.1 Current concepts in study design

Once the research question has been identified, the researcher must keep in mind the various limitations and biases affecting SRSs to reduce the likelihood of detecting spurious signals. Moreover, clinical, pharmacological, and statistical considerations are needed to select the most appropriate dataset, definition of cases, exposure, and covariables for stratification/adjustment.

Although the discussion on performance, accuracy, and reliability of different approaches to perform DAs was fascinating a decade ago, at present there is still no recognized *gold standard* methodology, and the key factor that may influence results is represented by the threshold defined for the number of cases [69, 70]. DAs in spontaneous reporting databases test whether an ADR is reported more frequently than expected; they allow identifying the so-called SDRs [23, 71]. These SDRs must be differentiated from safety signals because the existence of a SDR is not sufficient to constitute a safety signal (it does not always result in one, in fact), and a safety signal does not always imply a corresponding SDR [72].

As previously described, the various SRSs differ in terms of accessibility, catchment area, drug codification, and other technical issues. For instance, two key steps must be managed when analyzing the publicly available version of FAERS: drug mapping and removal of duplicates. These aspects have been extensively covered in the previous book chapter, and the reader should refer to this publication for details [73]. The FDA is continuously working to develop a probabilistic record-linkage algorithm combining structured and unstructured data (narratives) to improve the detection rate and accordingly reduce the occurrence of false positive signals [74].

7.2 Bias and strategies for their minimization

Before considering a potential causal relationship for a given identified SDR, main biases that affect signal detection from spontaneous reporting must be eliminated or at least mitigated. Notably, even after accounting for major bias, clinical association cannot be inferred from SRSs, and **channeling bias** (selective

Bias	Example	Underlying reason	Minimization strategy
Indication bias	Angiotensin Converting Enzyme (ACE) inhibitors showing signal of hypoglycemia.	These agents are largely used in diabetic patients.	Sensitivity analysis including only nondiabetic patients (i.e., using antidiabetic agents).
Drug competition bias	Anticoagulants when analyzing drug-induced bleeding.	Anticoagulants are expected to cause bleeding as toxic effect of their drug class.	Analysis by excluding reports with anticoagulants.
Event competition bias	Extrapyramidal syndrome (ES) when analyzing first-generation antipsychotics (FGA).	ES is a typical ADR in FGA-treated patients.	Analysis by excluding ES to detect new safety signal for FGA.
Notoriety bias	Rhabdomyolysis occurrence with statins after regulatory warnings.	After that alert, the number of events arose.	Studying signal before the alert.
Dilution bias	Suicide ideation related to new antidepressant.	A warning issued for a whole pharmacological class has stronger impact for newer drugs because the new ADR is diluted by other ADRs for older drugs.	Taking into account the time of drug approval and investigate different sources of dilution (e.g., warnings, publications, etc.).
Modified from [114].			

Table 3.
Major biases in disproportionality analyses and strategies for their minimization.

prescription of newer drugs to patients with more severe disease [75]) is unlikely to be fully accounted by statistical adjustments. They are described later together with practical examples and relevant minimization strategies as shown in **Table 3**.

Overall, we can identify: (A) **indication bias** when a drug is found to be associated with a given event for the sole reason that it is indicated in patients with comorbidities that increase the risk of that event; (B) **competition bias** also called "masking effect" when an event/drug more frequently reported for a given drug/event can "mask" identification of other possible ADRs/drugs [42, 76–82]; (C) **notoriety bias** when media attention (e.g., regulatory warning and milestone publication) causes over-reporting of peculiar ADR for specific drugs [37, 38]; and (D) **dilution bias** when a whole drug class is influenced by media attention for an event, older drugs with a larger numbers of reports are less likely to generate safety signal than newer drugs (with less reports) [83].

The **Weber effect** is an additional factor that may influence the reporting of given drugs, although it cannot be formally considered as a source of bias [84]. It was originally described as a higher reporting especially during the first 2 years after marketing approval, thus suggesting novelty *per se* as a risk factor for notification, although modern adverse event reporting systems seem less affected by this bias [43].

8. Unsettled issues

8.1 Patient reporting: current status

The 2012 PhV legislation forced national competent authorities and marketing authorization holders to record and report cases of suspected adverse reactions reported by patients [3]. This, in turn, caused legislation remarkable increase of the total number of patient reports (+113%) after 3 years, with the Netherlands, the UK, Germany, France, and Italy accounting for 75% of all patient reports [85]. The relevance of patient reports is heterogeneous, and a recent survey on 141 countries worldwide showed that in one-fourth of them, patients were not allowed to report. Conversely, countries receiving the highest percentage of patient reports in 2014 were the USA (64%) and Canada (30%).

More than 70 countries had fewer than 50 reports from patients [86]. The quality and the value of patient reports in the context of signal detection were evaluated in many published studies [87–91]. The value of the reports as a signal is directly dependent on the amount of clinically relevant information, in addition to the fact that an ADR report requires a thorough examination of the potential drug-event association. Most of the published studies comparing information reported by patients and healthcare professionals focused on the completeness of information [86, 92].

Patient reports give detailed descriptions of suspected ADRs, attribute reactions to specific medicines, and provide information useful for assessing causality. Patient reports often have richer narratives than those of healthcare professionals, including detailed information about the impact of the suspected ADR on the patient's life [91].

Many studies, mainly from the UK and the Netherlands, showed that patient reports allow for the identification of new ADRs and lead to the strengthening of signal detection activities [90, 93, 94].

In summary, patient's reporting offers a different perspective in drug safety assessment and may potentially contribute in signal detection. However, it is important to further investigate its actual role in drug safety assessment; in fact, the large number of reports without clear causal relationship (recently called "precautionary report") may alter adverse event profile by masking safety signals or, conversely, creating spurious associations [95].

8.2 Ethical and transparency issues

The relevance of patient reporting highlights the need of public access to spontaneous reporting data, and many countries now provide public access to SRSs, with the possibility to have summary presentations for reactions associated to each single drug in the database or a case listing of limited information for each single case report. Both EMA and WHO Uppsala Monitoring Centre (UMC) developed web tools to access a limited set of spontaneous reporting data in their database, EudraVigilance (adrreports.eu) and VigiBase (vigiaccess.org).

The EMA policy includes the possibility for academia or nonprofit organization to ask for a greater access to data as aggregated data outputs or line listings based on core data elements (http://www.ema.europa.eu/ema/index.jsp?curl=pages/regulation/general/general_content_000674.jsp). However, it has been commented that the EMA's approach to transparency over PhV data is too timid. The public access of PhV data is even more restricted for vaccines, mainly due to the potential negative impact of this public access to the vaccination campaigns. The reporting of serious adverse events not causally related to the vaccination could lead to a misrepresentation of vaccine risks that could be used by antivaccine movement. To our knowledge, very few European countries (e.g., Italy and the Netherlands) give public access to spontaneous data related to vaccines.

A different approach to transparency is followed by UMC and FDA. In VigiBase, custom search service provided by UMC is performed upon request. Any stakeholders can use the custom search services to request a limited set of data for specific studies or projects for a fee.

The best level of transparency is observed for FDA data. Data for both drugs (FAERS) and vaccine (VAERS) can be obtained using web-based search tools that return structured and/or unstructured data. Moreover, the entire database is quarterly downloadable in comma-separated value (CSV) or other formats. This access needs technical skills to properly process the relational database files and any unstructured fields. However, it gives the possibility to any users to analyze FDA spontaneous reporting data even applying DAs [5]. Since June 2014, the FDA developed an innovative platform called openFDA (openfda.gov) to facilitate access and use of big important FDA public datasets by developers, researchers, and the public through harmonization of data across disparate FDA datasets provided via application programming interfaces (APIs) [96]. Recently, the FDA has also launched the FAERS Public Dashboard, a highly interactive web-based tool that will allow to query FAERS data in a user-friendly fashion (https://fis.fda.gov/sense/app/777e9f4d-0cf8-448e-8068-f564c31baa25/sheet/7a47a261-d58b-4203-a8aa-6d3021737452/state/analysis). These different approaches to public access spontaneous reporting data lead to a bizarre situation because the reports included in EudraVigilance, VigiBase, and FAERS are largely overlapped, and it could be possible to have different information for the same report.

8.3 Social media: opportunities and challenges

An area of emerging interest for research is represented by the use of information provided by patients in social media on personal experiences when using a given drug. At present, it is under investigation whether or not (and how) social media data mining can contribute to signal detection [94, 95].

A recent review summarizes prevalence, frequency, and comparative value of information on adverse events of healthcare interventions from user comments and videos in social media. The study assessed over 174 social media sites, with discussion forums (71%) being the most popular. The overall prevalence of adverse event reports in social media varied from 0.2 to 8% of posts. Moreover, there was general agreement on overall concordance between adverse events mentioned in social media and those already documented in other sources (such as drug labels and published trials) [97].

The web-recognizing adverse drug reaction (Web-RADR) project, leaded by EMA and funded within the innovative medicines innovation (IMI), aims to recommend policies, frameworks, tools, and methodologies in the use of social media and mobile technology to improve drug safety [98]. Specific objectives are as follows: (a) to develop the specific mobile application prototypes to support adverse drug reaction reporting and the provision of drug safety information to application users and (b) to assess the usefulness of social media data for PhV and more specifically in signal detection activities.

The theoretical advantages of social media in the context of signal detection rely on potential earlier identification of rare and serious drug-related problems, in comparison with conventional SRSs, considering the opportunity to share information as fast as possible and the large number of active users in the social media. It has been reported that patient reports of suspected adverse reactions, particularly for specific reactions, can precede those of healthcare professionals [99]. One study of social media posts containing discussions of adverse drug events ("Proto-AEs") found that there were nearly three times as many Proto-AEs found in Twitter data than reported to the FDA by consumers, with rank correlation between them at the distribution of reactions at MedDRA SOC level [100].

Another important value from social media analyses comes from extracting qualitative insights into the actual discussions made by patients around a drug and an adverse event. This can be of great value for addressing issues related to the patient experience around an ADR and its impact on the quality of life [101]. Moreover, mining data from social media gives us a greater chance of capturing ADRs that a patient would not necessarily complain about to their doctor or nurse and can also help assessment of the risk perceptions of patients.

Key challenge is represented by the identification of drugs and ADRs in the text strings through a particular type of machine learning called natural language processing (NLP). From the perspective of PhV and NLP specifically, user posts on social media contain colloquial language and also misspellings. Especially when using lexicon-based approaches, these present problems as the accuracy of direct matches decreases. Colloquial and informal language is more difficult to parse, and thus, recent research tasks have focused on developing NLP tools specifically for data from social media [102, 103]. The balance between sensitivity and specificity of these tools in identifying ADRs is a key issue because a high number of false positives could heavily impact the efficacy of signal detection activities.

Another key element is the quality of the information on adverse events reported in the social media, which was analyzed only by a few works. A study where Internet narratives posted by patients were evaluated showed that the informativeness level was very incomplete and makes their assessment and use for PhV purpose difficult [104].

Concerning the potential of social media analyzes for earlier signal detection, contrasting data are published [105, 106].

Social media data mining uses information for PhV purposes, which were not primarily shared by the patient for this purpose. This raises a number of ethical questions, especially about identification of individuals by utilizing additional information, such as the geocode location on posting, username, and other potentially personally identifiable information [107], which are still unresolved. How would patient using social media react when approached for additional information by organizations that collect PhV data? Since this is a new area, ethically sound policy guidance needs to be developed.

A different approach in the use of Internet data for signal detection is the use of anonymized logs of web searchers [108]. In a recent study, a web-based search query method called "query log reaction score" was developed to detect whether adverse events associated with certain drugs could be found from search engine query data. The web query methods have moderate sensitivity (80%) in detecting signals in web query data compared with reference signal detection algorithms, but many false positives were generated, and this method had low specificity [109].

9. Future perspectives

The continuous increasing number of spontaneous reports and the increasing quality in their systematic archiving and accessing comply scientific community to improve methods of analysis and ways to interpret them for regulatory, clinical, and research purposes.

A specific debated issue on the current role of data-mining procedures of SRSs regards the possibility to directly compare drugs within the same therapeutic class [110]. We are in favor of this approach and strongly encourage further research regarding the use of SRSs, under stringently defined conditions, to compare adverse event rates for drugs [111]. To this aim, all the following criteria must be fulfilled:

1. *Same therapeutic indication(s)*. The effect of the underlying disease may be reduced by restricting DAs to drugs within the same therapeutic area [29, 30].

2. *Similar market penetration and utilization*. Drug consumption/prescription should be considered in order to: (i) complement DAs by highlighting possible risk differences through reporting rates (especially for vaccines and DMEs) [112]; (ii) weigh the drug risk at the population level (and assess the public health impact of ADRs); and (iii) prioritize safety signals emerging from traditional DAs [113].

3. *Similar time on the market*. This aspect should be carefully considered in the analyses to avoid the temporal or time-point bias, especially when comparing first- versus second-generation drugs. Standardization of the time on the market using the same fixed-length post-approval time-frame has been proposed [110].

4. *Data distortions are unlikely to occur or apply in a similar manner across the drugs under investigation*. Stratification (for age and sex) or adjustment should always be considered to minimize the presence of known confounders. Moreover, the existence of specific biases should be verified and accounted for.

An emerging application of SRSs, in the era of Big Data, is represented by their integration with other heterogeneous sources of healthcare data (e.g., the availability of prescription-data, hospital admission and discharge, population-based, disease-based, death registries, social media, and literature) to support proactive PhV in the risk-benefit assessment, as performed in the ARITMO projects through the Dempster-Shafer approach [59].

Finally, the question arises as to whether all disproportionality studies should be published in scientific journals. Supporters of scientific transparency and full release of datasets via Open Science would undoubtedly call for public availability of study results, including negative findings. A proposal was recently formulated [114].

This controversy on the quality of DAs raises the concern on how best assess it and reach consensus on a "set of minimum requirements to assess the quality of DAs in terms of study conception, performing and reporting." Provisional criteria have been recently proposed (from the experience of antidiabetic drugs) [114], but further discussion is warranted:

- **Clear title**. Avoid the general terms such as "pharmacovigilance analysis." Prefer the following terms: "disproportionality analysis," "analysis of spontaneous reporting system," and "analysis of spontaneous reports."

- **Scientifically sound study conception**. The scientific rationale must be clearly indicated and fall within one of these aforementioned categories (DAs are particularly suited for DMEs). Regulatory approach (i.e., identification of a potential signal during routine monitoring of spontaneous reporting systems) and commissioned analysis for regulatory purposes should not be formally eligible for publication in a journal, unless an added value emerges (e.g., the analysis is extended to the entire pharmacological class).

- **Transparent study design**. The unit of analysis should be described. Case(s) and exposure (reference group) definition should be specifically defined. The search strategy must be stated, and a clear description behind the choice is warranted. Key confounders to be accounted for must be *a priori* identified. Strategies to handle these biases must be indicated, including stratified or adjusted analyses. Notoriety must be carefully assessed: a structured literature evaluation is recommended, instead of a mere check to summary of product characteristics.

- **Balanced discussion and conclusion**. Prefer the term "disproportionality signal" and "signal of disproportionate reporting," and avoid the terms such as "alarm signal," "signal of risk," "increased risk," "association," "incidence." Compare the results with those emerging from similar studies (emerged from the structure literature evaluation). Limitations should be provided in a dedicated section, avoid a mere listing of known biases affecting spontaneous reporting system. Avoid the specific recommendations (decision-making approach) to support drug prescription or selection of drugs claimed to be safer.

From a technical standpoint, good signal detection practices have been published by the Innovative Medicines Initiative Pharmacoepidemiological Research on Outcomes of Therapeutics by a European ConsorTium (PROTECT) project, which have formulated 39 recommendations for those working in the PhV community [115].

A final issue regards the *timeliness* of publishing DAs when keeping with signal detection. For instance, the analysis by Elashoff et al. [16] on pancreatitis reports with incretin-based drugs, apart from methodological flaws and data misinterpretation causing unjustified alarm, was also untimely, considering that observational studies had already been carried out. Conversely, liver injury with direct-acting oral anticoagulants (DOACs) was studies because of limited predictivity of premarketing phases in detecting clinical signals of liver toxicity and previous concern with ximelagatran: the disproportionality signal raised for rivaroxaban in

FAERS [116] was tested by the recent US population-based studies, which found lower hospitalization rates for liver injury with DOAC initiators than patients starting warfarin, with rivaroxaban and dabigatran associated with the highest and lowest risk [117, 118], although confounders are likely to exist [119, 120]. This case underscores the value of performing well-conducted DAs and the importance of directing subsequent analytical research to confirm or refute the drug-related hypothesis.

All these unsettled issues witness the need and the importance of implementing research to finally clarify the role of DAs in clinical practice.

10. Concluding remarks

Regulators and especially clinicians are appreciating the importance and the role of DAs to monitor and assess the safety profile of marketed drugs. All "actors" dealing with SRSs must always be aware of the so-called seduction bias and self-deception bias (i.e., over-reliance on mathematical models and the subconscious confidence in expecting a given output from results), thus be reminded of inherent limitations that, at present, do not allow to assess actual risk in clinical practice, mainly because of the lack of certainty in the occurrence of adverse events and the lack of exposure data [121].

From a research perspective, there is an urgent need to raise the bar, aiming to increase the accuracy and reproducibility (in one word the quality) of this kind of study. From one side, there is a room for improvement in several aspects of the analysis of SRSs, including relevant implications and their appropriate use such as the aspect of "no findings" (i.e., findings of nondisproportional results), which has not received sufficient attention so far. Moreover, different research teams are implementing sophisticated methods to account for confounders in signal detection, so that DAs may approach relative risk. In the meantime, we propose to include disproportionality studies in (qualitative) systematic reviews keeping results separated from pooled risk estimates of (quantitative) meta-analyses [63].

In conclusion, SRSs represent an invaluable source to monitor and assess the safety of medications, including drugs, vaccines, and healthcare products.

We call for a responsible use and publication of DAs, which should be regulated through a consensus approach among experts; this would finally establish the use and transferability of DAs in clinical practice.

Author details

Emanuel Raschi[1], Ugo Moretti[2], Francesco Salvo[3,4,5], Antoine Pariente[3,4,5], Ippazio Cosimo Antonazzo[1], Fabrizio De Ponti[1] and Elisabetta Poluzzi[1*]

1 Department of Medical and Surgical Sciences, University of Bologna, Bologna, Italy

2 Department of Public Health and Community Medicine, University of Verona, Verona, Italy

3 University of Bordeaux, U657, Bordeaux, France

4 INSERM U657, Bordeaux, France

5 CIC Bordeaux CIC1401, Bordeaux, France

*Address all correspondence to: elisabetta.poluzzi@unibo.it

IntechOpen

References

[1] Edwards IR, Aronson JK. Adverse drug reactions: Definitions, diagnosis, and management. Lancet. 2000;**356**:1255-1259

[2] European Parliament. Regulation (EU) 1235/2010—2010 pharmacovigilance legislation. 2010. Available from: http://eur-lex.europa.eu/LexUriServ/LexUriServ.do?uri=OJ:L:2010:348:0001:0016:EN:PDF

[3] European Council (2010) Directive 2010/84/EU—2010 pharmacovigilance legislation. Available: http://eur-lex.europa.eu/LexUriServ/LexUriServ.do?uri=OJ:L:2010:348:0074:0099:EN:PDF

[4] Laporte JR. Fifty years of pharmacovigilance—Medicines safety and public health. Pharmacoepidemiology and Drug Safety. 2016;**25**:725-732

[5] Poluzzi E, Raschi E, Moretti U, De Ponti F. Drug-induced torsades de pointes: Data mining of the public version of the FDA adverse event reporting system (AERS). Pharmacoepidemiology and Drug Safety. 2009;**18**:512-518

[6] Poluzzi E, Raschi E, Motola D, Moretti U, De Ponti F. Antimicrobials and the risk of torsades de pointes: The contribution from data mining of the US FDA adverse event reporting system. Drug Safety. 2010;**33**:303-314

[7] Harpaz R, DuMouchel W, LePendu P, Bauer-Mehren A, Ryan P, Shah NH. Performance of pharmacovigilance signal-detection algorithms for the FDA adverse event reporting system. Clinical Pharmacology and Therapeutics. 2013;**93**:539-546

[8] Coloma PM, Trifiro G, Patadia V, Sturkenboom M. Postmarketing safety surveillance: Where does signal detection using electronic healthcare records fit into the big picture? Drug Safety. 2013;**36**:183-197

[9] Arnaud M, Begaud B, Thurin N, Moore N, Pariente A, Salvo F. Methods for safety signal detection in healthcare databases: A literature review. Expert Opinion on Drug Safety. 2017;**16**:721-732

[10] Anton R, Haas M, Arlett P, Weise M, Balabanov P, Mazzaglia G, et al. Drug-induced progressive multifocal leukoencephalopathy in multiple sclerosis: European regulators' perspective. Clinical Pharmacology and Therapeutics. 2017;**102**:283-289

[11] Dal Pan GJ, Arlett PR. The US Food and Drug Administration-European Medicines Agency collaboration in pharmacovigilance: Common objectives and common challenges. Drug Safety. 2015;**38**:13-15

[12] Pacurariu AC, Coloma PM, van HA, Genov G, Sturkenboom MC, Straus SM. A description of signals during the first 18 months of the EMA pharmacovigilance risk assessment committee. Drug Safety. 2014;**37**:1059-1066

[13] Pageot C, Bezin J, Smith A, Arnaud M, Salvo F, Haramburu F, et al. Impact of medicine withdrawal on reporting of adverse events involving therapeutic alternatives: A study from the French Spontaneous Reporting Database. Drug Safety. 2017;**40**:1099-1107

[14] Bohm R, von HL, Herdegen T, Klein HJ, Bruhn O, Petri H, et al. OpenVigil FDA—Inspection of U.S. American adverse drug events pharmacovigilance data and novel clinical applications. PLoS One. 2016;**11**:e0157753

[15] Sakaeda T, Tamon A, Kadoyama K, Okuno Y. Data mining of the public version of the FDA adverse event

reporting system. International Journal of Medical Sciences. 2013;**10**:796-803

[16] Elashoff M, Matveyenko AV, Gier B, Elashoff R, Butler PC. Pancreatitis, pancreatic, and thyroid cancer with glucagon-like peptide-1-based therapies. Gastroenterology. 2011;**141**:150-156

[17] Hauben M, Hung EY. Revisiting the reported signal of acute pancreatitis with rasburicase: An object lesson in pharmacovigilance. Therapeutic Advances in Drug Safety. 2016;7:94-101

[18] Hauben M, Hung EY, Hanretta KC, Bangalore S, Snow V. Safety of perflutren ultrasound contrast agents: A disproportionality analysis of the US FAERS database. Drug Safety. 2015;**38**:1127-1139

[19] Gagne JJ. Finding meaningful patterns in adverse drug event reports. JAMA Internal Medicine. 2014;**174**:1934-1935

[20] Greenblatt DJ. The pharmacovigilance syndrome. Journal of Clinical Psychopharmacology. 2015;**35**:361-363

[21] Onakpoya IJ, Heneghan CJ, Aronson JK. Post-marketing withdrawal of 462 medicinal products because of adverse drug reactions: A systematic review of the world literature. BMC Medicine. 2016;**14**:10

[22] Moore N, Blin P, Gulmez SE. New oral anticoagulants (NOAC) and liver injury. Journal of Hepatology. 2014;**61**:198-199

[23] Bate A, Evans SJ. Quantitative signal detection using spontaneous ADR reporting. Pharmacoepidemiology and Drug Safety. 2009;**18**:427-436

[24] de Boer A. When to publish measures of disproportionality derived from spontaneous reporting

databases? British Journal of Clinical Pharmacology. 2011;**72**:909-911

[25] Montastruc JL, Sommet A, Bagheri H, Lapeyre-Mestre M. Benefits and strengths of the disproportionality analysis for identification of adverse drug reactions in a pharmacovigilance database. British Journal of Clinical Pharmacology. 2011;**72**:905-908

[26] Giezen TJ, Mantel-Teeuwisse AK, Meyboom RH, Straus SM, Leufkens HG, Egberts TC. Mapping the safety profile of biologicals: A disproportionality analysis using the WHO adverse drug reaction database, VigiBase. Drug Safety. 2010;**33**:865-878

[27] Piccinni C, Motola D, Marchesini G, Poluzzi E. Assessing the association of pioglitazone use and bladder cancer through drug adverse event reporting. Diabetes Care. 2011;**34**:1369-1371

[28] Poluzzi E, Raschi E, Koci A, Moretti U, Spina E, Behr ER, et al. Antipsychotics and torsadogenic risk: Signals emerging from the US FDA adverse event reporting system database. Drug Safety. 2013;**36**:467-479

[29] Salvo F, Raschi E, Moretti U, Chiarolanza A, Fourrier-Reglat A, Moore N, et al. Pharmacological prioritisation of signals of disproportionate reporting: Proposal of an algorithm and pilot evaluation. European Journal of Clinical Pharmacology. 2014;**70**:617-625

[30] Grundmark B, Holmberg L, Garmo H, Zethelius B. Reducing the noise in signal detection of adverse drug reactions by standardizing the background: A pilot study on analyses of proportional reporting ratios-by-therapeutic area. European Journal of Clinical Pharmacology. 2014;**70**:627-635

[31] Raschi E, Poluzzi E, Koci A, Antonazzo IC, Marchesini G, De Ponti F. Dipeptidyl peptidase-4 inhibitors and

heart failure: Analysis of spontaneous reports submitted to the FDA adverse event reporting system. Nutrition, Metabolism, and Cardiovascular Diseases. 2016;**26**:380-386

[32] Raschi E, Parisotto M, Forcesi E, La Placa M, Marchesini G, De Ponti F, et al. Adverse events with sodium-glucose co-transporter-2 inhibitors: A global analysis of international spontaneous reporting systems. Nutrition, Metabolism, and Cardiovascular Diseases. 2017;**27**:1098-1107

[33] De Bruin ML, Pettersson M, Meyboom RH, Hoes AW, Leufkens HG. Anti-HERG activity and the risk of drug-induced arrhythmias and sudden death. European Heart Journal. 2005;**26**:590-597

[34] Montastruc F, Palmaro A, Bagheri H, Schmitt L, Montastruc JL, Lapeyre-Mestre M. Role of serotonin 5-HT2C and histamine H1 receptors in antipsychotic-induced diabetes: A pharmacoepidemiological-pharmacodynamic study in VigiBase. European Neuropsychopharmacology. 2015;**25**:1556-1565

[35] Nguyen TT, Pariente A, Montastruc JL, Lapeyre-Mestre M, Rousseau V, Rascol O, et al. An original pharmacoepidemiological-pharmacodynamic method: Application to antipsychotic-induced movement disorders. British Journal of Clinical Pharmacology. 2017;**83**:612-622

[36] Moore TJ, Glenmullen J, Mattison DR. Reports of pathological gambling, hypersexuality, and compulsive shopping associated with dopamine receptor agonist drugs. JAMA Internal Medicine. 2014;**174**:1930-1933

[37] Pariente A, Gregoire F, Fourrier-Reglat A, Haramburu F, Moore N. Impact of safety alerts on measures of disproportionality in spontaneous

reporting databases: The notoriety bias. Drug Safety. 2007;**30**:891-898

[38] Raschi E, Piccinni C, Poluzzi E, Marchesini G, De Ponti F. The association of pancreatitis with antidiabetic drug use: Gaining insight through the FDA pharmacovigilance database. Acta Diabetologica. 2013;**50**:569-577

[39] Hoffman KB, Demakas AR, Dimbil M, Tatonetti NP, Erdman CB. Stimulated reporting: The impact of US food and drug administration-issued alerts on the adverse event reporting system (FAERS). Drug Safety. 2014;**37**:971-980

[40] Maignen F, Hauben M, Hung E, Van HL, Dogne JM. Assessing the extent and impact of the masking effect of disproportionality analyses on two spontaneous reporting systems databases. Pharmacoepidemiology and Drug Safety. 2014;**23**:195-207

[41] Maignen F, Hauben M, Hung E, Holle LV, Dogne JM. A conceptual approach to the masking effect of measures of disproportionality. Pharmacoepidemiology and Drug Safety. 2014;**23**:208-217

[42] Arnaud M, Salvo F, Ahmed I, Robinson P, Moore N, Begaud B, et al. A method for the minimization of competition bias in signal detection from spontaneous reporting databases. Drug Safety. 2016;**39**:251-260

[43] Hoffman KB, Dimbil M, Erdman CB, Tatonetti NP, Overstreet BM. The Weber effect and the United States Food and Drug Administration's adverse event reporting system (FAERS): Analysis of sixty-two drugs approved from 2006 to 2010. Drug Safety. 2014;**37**:283-294

[44] Van Puijenbroek EP, Egberts AC, Heerdink ER, Leufkens HG. Detecting drug-drug interactions using a

database for spontaneous adverse drug reactions: An example with diuretics and non-steroidal anti-inflammatory drugs. European Journal of Clinical Pharmacology. 2000;**56**:733-738

[45] Thakrar BT, Grundschober SB, Doessegger L. Detecting signals of drug-drug interactions in a spontaneous reports database. British Journal of Clinical Pharmacology. 2007;**64**:489-495

[46] Leone R, Magro L, Moretti U, Cutroneo P, Moschini M, Motola D, et al. Identifying adverse drug reactions associated with drug-drug interactions: Data mining of a spontaneous reporting database in Italy. Drug Safety. 2010;**33**:667-675

[47] Strandell J, Wahlin S. Pharmacodynamic and pharmacokinetic drug interactions reported to VigiBase, the WHO global individual case safety report database. European Journal of Clinical Pharmacology. 2011;**67**:633-641

[48] Labat V, Arnaud M, Miremont-Salame G, Salvo F, Begaud B, Pariente A. Risk of myopathy associated with DPP-4 inhibitors in combination with statins: A disproportionality analysis using data from the WHO and French Spontaneous Reporting Databases. Diabetes Care. 2017;**40**:e27-e29

[49] Strandell J, Caster O, Bate A, Noren N, Edwards IR. Reporting patterns indicative of adverse drug interactions: A systematic evaluation in VigiBase. Drug Safety. 2011;**34**:253-266

[50] Fadini GP, Bonora BM, Mayur S, Rigato M, Avogaro A. Dipeptidyl peptidase-4 inhibitors moderate the risk of genitourinary tract infections associated with sodium-glucose co-transporter-2 inhibitors. Diabetes, Obesity & Metabolism. 2018;**20**:740-744

[51] Fadini GP, Sarangdhar M, Avogaro A. Pharmacovigilance evaluation of the association between DPP-4 inhibitors and heart failure: Stimulated reporting and moderation by drug interactions. Diabetes Therapy. 2018;**9**:851-861

[52] Dias P, Penedones A, Alves C, Ribeiro CF, Marques FB. The role of disproportionality analysis of pharmacovigilance databases in safety regulatory actions: A systematic review. Current Drug Safety. 2015;**10**:234-250

[53] Hochberg AM, Hauben M. Time-to-signal comparison for drug safety data-mining algorithms vs. traditional signaling criteria. Clinical Pharmacology and Therapeutics. 2009;**85**:600-606

[54] Ralph EI. Causality assessment in pharmacovigilance: Still a challenge. Drug Safety. 2017;**40**:365-372

[55] Agbabiaka TB, Savovic J, Ernst E. Methods for causality assessment of adverse drug reactions: A systematic review. Drug Safety. 2008;**31**:21-37

[56] Sassolas B, Haddad C, Mockenhaupt M, Dunant A, Liss Y, Bork K, et al. ALDEN, an algorithm for assessment of drug causality in Stevens-Johnson syndrome and toxic epidermal necrolysis: Comparison with case-control analysis. Clinical Pharmacology and Therapeutics. 2010;**88**:60-68

[57] Garcia-Cortes M, Stephens C, Lucena MI, Fernandez-Castaner A, Andrade RJ. Causality assessment methods in drug induced liver injury: Strengths and weaknesses. Journal of Hepatology. 2011;**55**:683-691

[58] van Eekeren R, Rolfes L, Koster AS, Magro L, Parthasarathi G, Al Ramimmy H, et al. What future healthcare professionals need to know about pharmacovigilance: Introduction of the WHO PV core curriculum for university teaching with focus on clinical aspects.

Drug Safety. 2018. DOI: 10.1007/s40264-018-0681-z

[59] Final Report Summary-ARITMO (Arrhythmogenic potential of Drugs)—Project ID: 241679—Funded under FP7-HEALTH. 2017. Available from: http://cordis.europa.eu/result/rcn/141814_en.html

[60] Park SJ, Ogunseitan OA, Lejano RP. Dempster-Shafer theory applied to regulatory decision process for selecting safer alternatives to toxic chemicals in consumer products. Integrated Environmental Assessment and Management. 2014;10:12-21

[61] Li Y, Ryan PB, Wei Y, Friedman C. A method to combine signals from spontaneous reporting systems and observational healthcare data to detect adverse drug reactions. Drug Safety. 2015;38:895-908

[62] Pacurariu AC, Straus SM, Trifiro G, Schuemie MJ, Gini R, Herings R, et al. Useful interplay between spontaneous ADR reports and electronic healthcare records in signal detection. Drug Safety. 2015;38:1201-1210

[63] Gough G, Oliver S, Thomas J. An Introduction to Systematic Reviews. 2012. Available from: http://ec.europa.eu/health/ph_projects/2001/monitoring/fp_monitoring_2001_exs_12_en.pdf (First: 1-288)

[64] Cheng YJ, Nie XY, Chen XM, Lin XX, Tang K, Zeng WT, et al. The role of macrolide antibiotics in increasing cardiovascular risk. Journal of the American College of Cardiology. 2015;66:2173-2184

[65] Raschi E, Salvo F, Poluzzi E, De Ponti F. Safety meta-analysis: A call for appropriate use of disproportionality measures from spontaneous reporting systems. Journal of the American College of Cardiology. 2016;67:2193

[66] Khouri C, Lepelley M, Roustit M, Montastruc F, Humbert M, Cracowski JL. Comparative safety of drugs targeting the nitric oxide pathway in pulmonary hypertension: A mixed approach combining a meta-analysis of clinical trials and a disproportionality analysis from the World Health Organization Pharmacovigilance Database. Chest. 2017;S0012-3692(17):33265-33268

[67] Wald NJ, Morris JK. Teleoanalysis: Combining data from different types of study. British Medical Journal. 2003;327:616-618

[68] Macia-Martinez MA, de Abajo FJ, Roberts G, Slattery J, Thakrar B, Wisniewski AF. An empirical approach to explore the relationship between measures of disproportionate reporting and relative risks from analytical studies. Drug Safety. 2016;39:29-43

[69] Slattery J, Alvarez Y, Hidalgo A. Choosing thresholds for statistical signal detection with the proportional reporting ratio. Drug Safety. 2013;36:687-692

[70] Candore G, Juhlin K, Manlik K, Thakrar B, Quarcoo N, Seabroke S, et al. Comparison of statistical signal detection methods within and across spontaneous reporting databases. Drug Safety. 2015;38:577-587

[71] Van Puijenbroek EP, Bate A, Leufkens HG, Lindquist M, Orre R, Egberts AC. A comparison of measures of disproportionality for signal detection in spontaneous reporting systems for adverse drug reactions. Pharmacoepidemiology and Drug Safety. 2002;11:3-10

[72] Hauben M, Reich L, Gerrits CM, Younus M. Illusions of objectivity and a recommendation for reporting data mining results. European Journal of Clinical Pharmacology. 2007;63:517-521

[73] Poluzzi E, Raschi E, Piccinni C, De Ponti F. Data mining techniques in pharmacovigilance: Analysis of the publicly accessible FDA adverse event reporting system (AERS). In: Karahoca A, editor. Data Mining Applications in Engineering and Medicine. Croatia: InTech; 2012. pp. 265-302

[74] Kreimeyer K, Menschik D, Winiecki S, Paul W, Barash F, Woo EJ, et al. Using probabilistic record linkage of structured and unstructured data to identify duplicate cases in spontaneous adverse event reporting systems. Drug Safety. 2017;**40**:571-582

[75] Petri H, Urquhart J. Channeling bias in the interpretation of drug effects. Statistics in Medicine. 1991;**10**:577-581

[76] Gould AL. Practical pharmacovigilance analysis strategies. Pharmacoepidemiology and Drug Safety. 2003;**12**:559-574

[77] Almenoff J, Tonning JM, Gould AL, Szarfman A, Hauben M, Ouellet-Hellstrom R, et al. Perspectives on the use of data mining in pharmaco-vigilance. Drug Safety. 2005;**28**:981-1007

[78] Wang HW, Hochberg AM, Pearson RK, Hauben M. An experimental investigation of masking in the US FDA adverse event reporting system database. Drug Safety. 2010;**33**:1117-1133

[79] Pariente A, Didailler M, Avillach P, Miremont-Salame G, Fourrier-Reglat A, Haramburu F, et al. A potential competition bias in the detection of safety signals from spontaneous reporting databases. Pharmacoepidemiology and Drug Safety. 2010;**19**:1166-1171

[80] Pariente A, Avillach P, Salvo F, Thiessard F, Miremont-Salame G, Fourrier-Reglat A, et al. Effect of competition bias in safety signal generation: Analysis of a research database of spontaneous reports in France. Drug Safety. 2012;**35**:855-864

[81] Juhlin K, Ye X, Star K, Noren GN. Outlier removal to uncover patterns in adverse drug reaction surveillance—A simple unmasking strategy. Pharmacoepidemiology and Drug Safety. 2013;**22**:1119-1129

[82] Salvo F, Leborgne F, Thiessard F, Moore N, Begaud B, Pariente A. A potential event-competition bias in safety signal detection: Results from a spontaneous reporting research database in France. Drug Safety. 2013;**36**:565-572

[83] Pariente A, Daveluy A, Laribiere-Benard A, Miremont-Salame G, Begaud B, Moore N. Effect of date of drug marketing on disproportionality measures in pharmacovigilance: The example of suicide with SSRIs using data from the UK MHRA. Drug Safety. 2009;**32**:441-447

[84] Hartnell NR, Wilson JP. Replication of the Weber effect using postmarketing adverse event reports voluntarily submitted to the United States Food and Drug Administration. Pharmacotherapy. 2004;**24**:743-749

[85] Banovac M, Candore G, Slattery J, Houyez F, Haerry D, Genov G, et al. Patient reporting in the EU: Analysis of Eudravigilance Data. Drug Safety. 2017;**40**:629-645

[86] Matos C, Harmark L, van HF. Patient reporting of adverse drug reactions: An international survey of national competent authorities' views and needs. Drug Safety. 2016;**39**:1105-1116

[87] Inacio P, Cavaco A, Airaksinen M. The value of patient reporting to the pharmacovigilance system: A systematic review. British Journal of Clinical Pharmacology. 2017;**83**:227-246

[88] Avery AJ, Anderson C, Bond CM, Fortnum H, Gifford A, Hannaford PC, et al. Evaluation of patient reporting of adverse drug reactions to the UK 'Yellow Card Scheme': Literature review, descriptive and qualitative analyses, and questionnaire surveys. Health Technology Assessment. 2011;**15**:1-234

[89] Inch J, Watson MC, nakwe-Umeh S. Patient versus healthcare professional spontaneous adverse drug reaction reporting: A systematic review. Drug Safety. 2012;**35**:807-818

[90] van HF, de WS, Harmark L. The contribution of direct patient reported ADRs to drug safety signals in the Netherlands from 2010 to 2015. Pharmacoepidemiology and Drug Safety. 2017;**26**:977-983

[91] Rolfes L, van HF, van der LL, Taxis K, van PE. The quality of clinical information in adverse drug reaction reports by patients and healthcare professionals: A retrospective comparative analysis. Drug Safety. 2017;**40**:607-614

[92] Rolfes L, van HF, Wilkes S, van GK, van PE. Adverse drug reaction reports of patients and healthcare professionals-differences in reported information. Pharmacoepidemiology and Drug Safety. 2015;**24**:152-158

[93] Hazell L, Cornelius V, Hannaford P, Shakir S, Avery AJ. How do patients contribute to signal detection?: A retrospective analysis of spontaneous reporting of adverse drug reactions in the UK's Yellow Card Scheme. Drug Safety. 2013;**36**:199-206

[94] Watson S, Chandler RE, Taavola H, Harmark L, Grundmark B, Zekarias A, et al. Safety concerns reported by patients identified in a collaborative signal detection workshop using VigiBase: Results and reflections from Lareb and Uppsala Monitoring Centre. Drug Safety. 2017;**41**:203-212

[95] Klein K, Scholl JH, De Bruin ML, Van Puijenbroek EP, Leufkens HG, Stolk P. When more is less—An exploratory study of the precautionary reporting bias and its impact on safety signal detection. Clinical Pharmacology and Therapeutics. 2017;**103**: 296-303

[96] Kass-Hout TA, Xu Z, Mohebbi M, Nelsen H, Baker A, Levine J, et al. OpenFDA: An innovative platform providing access to a wealth of FDA's publicly available data. Journal of the American Medical Informatics Association. 2016;**23**:596-600

[97] Golder S, Norman G, Loke YK. Systematic review on the prevalence, frequency and comparative value of adverse events data in social media. British Journal of Clinical Pharmacology. 2015;**80**:878-888

[98] Ghosh R, Lewis D. Aims and approaches of Web-RADR: A consortium ensuring reliable ADR reporting via mobile devices and new insights from social media. Expert Opinion on Drug Safety. 2015;**14**:1845-1853

[99] Egberts TC, Smulders M, de Koning FH, Meyboom RH, Leufkens HG. Can adverse drug reactions be detected earlier? A comparison of reports by patients and professionals. British Medical Journal. 1996;**313**:530-531

[100] Freifeld CC, Brownstein JS, Menone CM, Bao W, Filice R, Kass-Hout T, et al. Digital drug safety surveillance: Monitoring pharmaceutical products in twitter. Drug Safety. 2014;**37**: 343-350

[101] Abou TM, Rossard C, Cantaloube L, Bouscaren N, Roche G, Pochard L, et al. Analysis of patients' narratives posted on social media websites on benfluorex's (Mediator(R)) withdrawal in France. Journal of Clinical Pharmacy and Therapeutics. 2014;**39**:53-55

[102] Nikfarjam A, Sarker A, O'Connor K, Ginn R, Gonzalez G. Pharmacovigilance from social media: Mining adverse drug reaction mentions using sequence labeling with word embedding cluster features. Journal of the American Medical Informatics Association. 2015;**22**:671-681

[103] Demner-Fushman D, Elhadad N. Aspiring to unintended consequences of natural language processing: A review of recent developments in clinical and consumer-generated text processing. Yearbook of Medical Informatics. 2016:224-233

[104] Kheloufi F, Default A, Blin O, Micallef J. Investigating patient narratives posted on Internet and their informativeness level for pharmacovigilance purpose: The example of comments about statins. Thérapie. 2017;**72**:483-490

[105] Pierce CE, Bouri K, Pamer C, Proestel S, Rodriguez HW, Van LH, et al. Evaluation of facebook and twitter monitoring to detect safety signals for medical products: An analysis of recent FDA safety alerts. Drug Safety. 2017;**40**:317-331

[106] Duh MS, Cremieux P, Audenrode MV, Vekeman F, Karner P, Zhang H, et al. Can social media data lead to earlier detection of drug-related adverse events? Pharmacoepidemiology and Drug Safety. 2016;**25**:1425-1433

[107] Sloane R, Osanlou O, Lewis D, Bollegala D, Maskell S, Pirmohamed M. Social media and pharmacovigilance: A review of the opportunities and challenges. British Journal of Clinical Pharmacology. 2015;**80**:910-920

[108] White RW, Wang S, Pant A, Harpaz R, Shukla P, Sun W, et al. Early identification of adverse drug reactions from search log data. Journal of Biomedical Informatics. 2016;**59**:42-48

[109] Colilla S, Tov EY, Zhang L, Kurzinger ML, Tcherny-Lessenot S, Penfornis C, et al. Validation of new signal detection methods for web query log data compared to signal detection algorithms used with FAERS. Drug Safety. 2017;**40**:399-408

[110] Michel C, Scosyrev E, Petrin M, Schmouder R. Can disproportionality analysis of post-marketing case reports be used for comparison of drug safety profiles? Clinical Drug Investigation. 2017;**37**:415-422

[111] Hochberg AM, Pearson RK, O'Hara DJ, Reisinger SJ. Drug-versus-drug adverse event rate comparisons: A pilot study based on data from the US FDA adverse event reporting system. Drug Safety. 2009;**32**:137-146

[112] Svendsen K, Halvorsen KH, Vorren S, Samdal H, Garcia B. Adverse drug reaction reporting: How can drug consumption information add to analyses using spontaneous reports? European Journal of Clinical Pharmacology. 2018;**74**:497-504

[113] Raschi E, De Ponti F. Drug utilization research and pharmacovigilance. In: Elsevier M, Wettermek B, Almarsdóttir AB, Andersen M, Benko R, Bennie M, Eriksson I, Godman B, Krska J, Poluzzi E, Taxis K, Vlahovic-Palcevski V, Stichele RV, editors. Drug Utilization Research: Methods and Applications. Chichester, UK: John Wiley & Sons; 2016

[114] Raschi E, Poluzzi E, Salvo F, Pariente A, De Ponti F, Marchesini G, et al. Pharmacovigilance of sodium-glucose co-transporter-2 inhibitors: What a clinician should know on disproportionality analysis of spontaneous reporting systems. Nutrition, Metabolism, and Cardiovascular Diseases. 2018;**28**:533-542

[115] Wisniewski AF, Bate A, Bousquet C, Brueckner A, Candore G, Juhlin K, et al. Good signal detection practices: Evidence from IMI PROTECT. Drug Safety. 2016;**39**:469-490

[116] Raschi E, Poluzzi E, Koci A, Salvo F, Pariente A, Biselli M, et al. Liver injury with novel oral anticoagulants: Assessing post-marketing reports in the US Food and Drug Administration adverse event reporting system. British Journal of Clinical Pharmacology. 2015;**80**:285-293

[117] Alonso A, MacLehose RF, Chen LY, Bengtson LG, Chamberlain AM, Norby FL, et al. Prospective study of oral anticoagulants and risk of liver injury in patients with atrial fibrillation. Heart. 2017;**103**:834-839

[118] Douros A, Azoulay L, Yin H, Suissa S, Renoux C. Non-vitamin K antagonist oral anticoagulants and risk of serious liver injury. Journal of the American College of Cardiology. 2018;**71**:1105-1113

[119] Alonso A, MacLehose RF, Chen LY, Bengtson LGS, Chamberlain AM, Norby FL, et al. Oral anticoagulants and liver injury: The threat of uncontrolled confounding. Heart. 2018;**104**:84

[120] Raschi E, De Ponti F. Liver injury with direct-acting anticoagulants: Has the fog cleared? Heart. 2017;**103**:2010

[121] Hauben M, Patadia V, Gerrits C, Walsh L, Reich L. Data mining in pharmacovigilance: The need for a balanced perspective. Drug Safety. 2005;**28**:835-842

Chapter 3

Pharmacovigilance in Pediatric Population

Roxana De Las Salas and Claudia Margarita Vásquez Soto

Abstract

Pharmacology in pediatric population has specific needs in pharmacovigilance. The lack of studies in children leads mostly to "off-label" prescribing and to an increased frequency of adverse drug reactions. Additionally, younger ages, male sex, prolonged and previous hospitalization, indication of antibiotics, and the number of prescribed drugs are factors associated with a higher risk of ADRs. Consequently, ADRs represent an additional burden of morbidity. This chapter will be focused on the most common adverse drug reactions in children (including infants and newborns), challenges, and new legislative tools in pediatric pharmacovigilance by using the Word Health Organization global individual case safety report database (VigiAccess) and results from a Latin American study.

Keywords: adverse drug reaction, child, pharmacoepidemiology

1. Introduction

The safety of medicines in children is a worldwide problem, and the pharmacological characteristics of infants require a specific knowledge by health-care professionals. In other words, to care for children, more training and expertise are necessary. Likewise, the lack of clinical trials in which children are included and the off-label use of medications are determining factors for having more adverse drug reactions than usually. In ambulatory and hospital settings, it is necessary to have personnel with training in taking care of children.

Pharmacovigilance (PV), as was mentioned in the other chapter, "is defined as the science and activities relating to the detection, assessment, understanding and prevention of adverse effects or any other drug-related problem" [1]. It is also proper to ensure that PV was born recently with the thalidomide disaster, with effects on children.

Considering the abovementioned, this chapter shows the main concepts of pharmacovigilance applied to the pediatric population and gives an idea of the main safety concerns of drugs used in the neonatology and pediatric wards and the most frequent adverse reactions. On the other hand, this adds new legislative tools in pediatric pharmacovigilance.

2. A brief history of the beginning of pharmacovigilance in pediatrics

The first example of a safety issue that led to a pharmacovigilance reflection was published in the British Medical Journal in 1877 by chloroform issues. The second problem happened in 1898 with the commercialization of diacetylmorphine, named as heroin, which started to be addictive at the beginning of the 1910s (500,000 dependent patients reported only in the US) [2]. In 1937, the use of diethylene glycol to solubilize sulfanilamide, without any toxic test previously studied, with a series 34 children deaths from kidney failure (of 103 cases) [3]. The third one was at the beginning of the 1950s (1954), diiododiethyl of tin was added to Stalinon®, a topical skin product, resulting in 102 cases of deaths associated with encephalopathy, and a hundred patients developed severe, irreversible, neurological aftereffects [2].

During the 1960s, many children were born with phocomelia and agenesis of the limbs as a side effect of thalidomide. Thalidomide was marketed in 1957 as an over-the-counter (OTC) hypnotic/sedative and a safe drug, later used in order to manage nausea in pregnant women. In 1961, Widukind Lenz, a German geneticist, linked the serious effects to the use of thalidomide during a congress. This was later confirmed in the same year by William McBride, who established a 20% of rise in phocomelia and agenesis of the limbs malformation. The results were more than 12,000 cases of teratogenic effects in children (not only limbs malformation) [2].

In response to the thalidomide disaster, the World Health Organization (WHO) formerly established its Program for International Drug Monitoring in 1968. In 1978, it is founded the Uppsala Monitoring Centre, a WHO collaborating center created in order to support the mentioned program.

Therefore, a new era of pharmacovigilance was initiated by children's big issues related to teratogenic effects. In other words, PV was born as a result of a disaster in children.

3. Key concepts of pharmacovigilance in pediatrics

According to the World Health Organization (WHO), an adverse drug reaction (ADR) is "a response to a drug which is noxious and unintended and which occurs at doses normally used in man for prophylaxis, diagnosis, or therapy of disease, or the modification of physiological function" [4].

In Spain, the pharmacovigilance system defines an ADR as any harmful and unintentional response to a medication. It not only includes harmful and involuntary effects derived from the authorized use of a medicine in normal doses but is also related to medication errors and off-label terms of the marketing authorization, including misuse, overdose, and abuse of the drug [5]. Terms such as side effect, adverse effect, undesirable effect, and collateral effect are synonymous of ADR.

The variability among pediatric population is associated with higher susceptibility for ADRs. Considering this, whenever there is an ADR, it is necessary to take into account not only the weight, height, and information of the medication but also the exact age of the child. For that reason, it is important to know the pharmacological differences in infants, as shown in **Table 1** [6, 7].

3.1 Challenges of pharmacovigilance in pediatrics

Despite international authorities' efforts to stimulate the notification of adverse drug reactions (ADRs), under-reporting is still quite common [8]. In part, this happens due to the voluntary notification system mainly. Other reasons could be related to problems with the ADR diagnosis, work overload of staff, and possible conflicts of interest [9]. Thereby, the most important challenges in PV are focused on those issues.

Despite the European Medicines Agency, Pharmacovigilance Risk Assessment Committee (PRAC) has a pediatric Committee (PDCO) that revise "all aspects of the risk management of the use of medicinal products"; and generate

Physiologic characteristics	Characteristics
Absorption	
Gastric pH	Lower bioavailability of weak acid drugs
	Higher bioavailability of weak bases
Gastrointestinal motility	Delayed absorption
Percutaneous absorption	Higher bioavailability
Muscle absorption	Variable (unknown)
Distribution	
Body water	Higher volume of distribution for hydrophilic drugs
	Less volume of distribution for hydrophilic drugs
Protein binding	Higher free fraction of drugs
Metabolism	
Phase I enzyme (cytochrome (CYP) P450)	Less hepatic clearance
Phase II enzyme (UGT)	Less hepatic clearance. Glucuronidation does not reach adult levels for at least 3 years of age
Elimination	
Renal excretion GFR (tubular absorption and secretion)	Lower renal clearance. Nephrogenesis is complete at 34 weeks of gestation. GFR reaches adult levels by 2 years of age

GFR, glomerular filtration rate; UGT, UDP-glucuronosyltransferase. Source: [6, 7].

Table 1.
Pharmacological characteristics that can condition the appearance of adverse reactions to medications.

recommendations of safety use of medicine in pediatrics, actually there are many challenges [10].

Intensive pharmacovigilance is needed in pediatric population, due to increased susceptibility to ADRs and predisposing factors [11, 12]. Intensive pharmacovigilance is defined as "the systematic monitoring of the occurrence of adverse events resulting from drug use during the entire length of prescription" [13]. This is the first pharmacovigilance challenge, to achieve integration in health systems in a proactive and routinary way. The truth is that pharmacovigilance must function dynamically and based on the fundamental pillars of public health: protection, promotion, and prevention.

Another important challenge is to implement a mandatory reporting system, because in the case of adverse reactions in children, it is always important to analyze the reason for ADR. This is perhaps the most important challenge.

In addition, as shown in **Image 1**, to achieve a benefit-risk balance in pediatric populations, it is necessary to implement a dynamic PV cycle that allows the gain of knowledge and the management of risks associated with medicines in children. That could be an important new legislative tool in pediatric pharmacovigilance.

On the other hand, due to off-label being permitted, authorities have to demand from pharmacy industry the inclusion of children in clinical trial. The main reason for that is that if it is not ethical to include children in clinical trials, much less is to use a medicine that has never been prescribed or used in children population before.

Despite, PRAC-PDCO is constantly communicating about the importance of ADR monitoring and reporting suspected ADR in order to create signals for pediatric population. Some legislative tools for improving pharmacovigilance in pediatric population could be to promote research networks and ADR report in children (including pregnancy), to create networks of pediatric use of medicine and pharmacovigilance, to pilot new approaches to strengthen signal detection, to work on medication error, and to create a PRAC-PDCO collaborative working on benefit-risk worldwide [10] (**Image 2**).

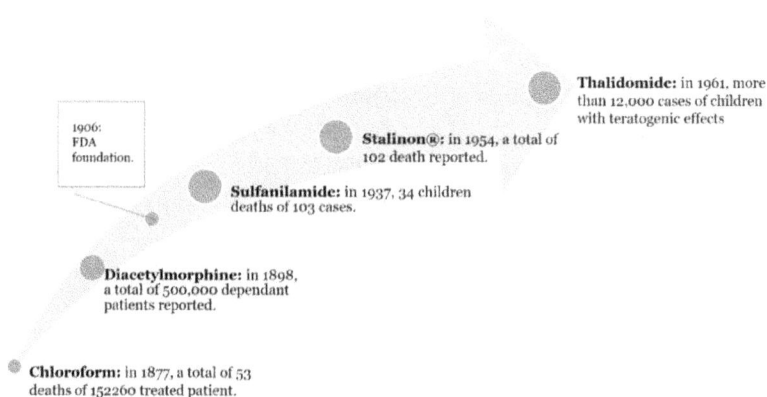

Image 1.
Significant milestones of the history of pharmacovigilance in pediatrics.

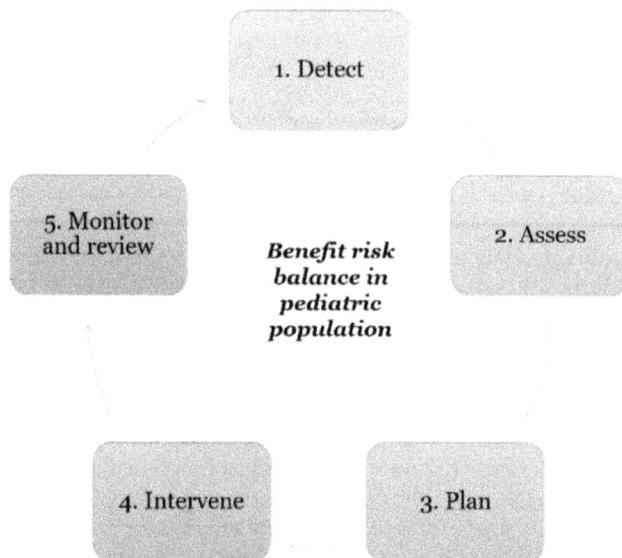

Image 2.
Pharmacovigilance cycle. Source: Taken from: Raine J. Pharmacovigilance in Paediatric Population. The PRAC's perspective EU: EMA; 2014. (10).

3.2 Importance of pharmacovigilance in children's intensive care units

Patient safety in child intensive care units is a priority in health care, in which the entire interdisciplinary team has to use guidelines and protocols that attempt to minimize the errors that occur in clinical practice. These controls can be efficient and effective, but sometimes fail, and it produces an error during the prescribing or the administration of medications [14]. Due to complex diseases, critically ill children (newborns and infants) in intensive care units are in a higher risk of developing ADRs [15].

In the neonatal and pediatric intensive care units, efforts have been made to strengthen drug administration processes focused on improving patient identification, drug, and dosage, through a list of checkups with a clear and timely focus on risk management in the use of medications [14].

Therefore, as a component of patient safety policy, in each health institution, this must be effectively coordinated with the pharmacovigilance system; although what this policy is looking for and working for is the patient safety, seen from the integral clinical component and from the pharmacovigilance perspective, the medicine and its use are taken as the central axis. Therefore, the need to efficiently regulate both actions is emphasized, with the aim of not affecting the duplication of efforts and results, in order to achieve maximum patient safety and the most optimal management possible on the safe use of medicines [16].

Due to ADR and inadequate practices on the use of medications which make up a large percentage of hospital admissions and extensive hospital days of stay, it is vitally important to have active pharmacovigilance, improving the education and communication of all risks related to medications. All health teams have to use the same language, and this is possible because the protocols and clinical guidelines established in the institutions, as well as improving the notification of errors in order to analyze and to improve plans [17].

4. Adverse drug reactions in children

The WHO Global Individual Case Safety Report (ICSR) database (VigiBase®), using spontaneous notification system, has reported ADR rates of 7.7% (268.145) in children from 0 to 17 years of age [18]. Nevertheless, ADR prevalence in children can vary due to patient characteristics, methodology used in the evaluation of the suspected ADR, and pharmacological treatments. In addition, ADR only can be classified as definitive if the medication or placebo was readministered and the blood concentration of the drug measured, which is not possible, even for ethical issues in the care of children.

Country/ study	Study ID	ADR incidence	Age	Type of study	Number of patients	Type of service
Spain	Belen 2016 [19]	17.00%	≤29 days (neonates)	Prospective cohort study	332	Neonatal ward
Mexico	Vásquez-Alvarez 2017 [20]	1.75%	≤18 years of age	Prospective cross-sectional	1083	Hospital admissions
Colombia	De las salas 2016 [21, 22]	21.31%	≤5 years of age	Prospective cohort study	1056	Neonatal and pediatrics wards
Brazil	Barbosa 2006 [23]	12.50%	≤16 years of age	Prospective cohort study	265	Pediatric ward
United States*	Sharek 2006 [24]	4.54%	≤29 days (neonates)	Retrospective cross-sectional study	749	NICUs
India	Digra 2015 [25]	0.36%	≤19	Prospective observational study	28,864	Pediatric ward

*Included one Canada neonatal care unit of 15. NICU, neonatal intensive care unit.

Table 2.
Incidence of ADR in children from different countries around the world.

Age/drug	Ibuprofen	ASA*	Diclofenac	Naproxen	Indomethacin	Piroxicam
0–27 days	416	122	53	36	180	9
28 days to 23 months	3113	533	195	263	107	16
2–11 years	12,428	2196	986	922	144	67
12–17 years	6016	1741	2091	1622	231	184
Total	21,973	4592	3325	2843	662	276

Source: vigiaccess.org. Accessed: 08-15-2018.
Acetylsalicylic acid. NSAIDs, nonsteroidal anti-inflammatory drugs.

Table 3.
NSAID ADRs in children.

Many studies conducted in different countries, using mostly prospective observational studies, have reported ADR rates ranging from 0.36 to 21.31%. This is described in **Table 2**.

4.1 Individual case safety report

Considering the importance of ADR notifications reported to the Uppsala Monitoring Centre (UMC), some of the drugs with greater frequency of use or with relevant aspects of safety in children have been selected. As nonsteroidal anti-inflammatory drugs (NSAIDs), anticonvulsant, opioids, and certain cold medicines are frequently used and have relevant issues in medicine safety in children, this section presents the results of the World Health Organization global individual case safety report database (VigiAccess).

The ADR frequency report for NSAIDs is variable. Ibuprofen is the drug with the highest ADR report in children. It could be due to the fact that it is one of the most used drugs in this population. The comparison of other NSAID ADRs is presented in **Table 3**.

Different studies [26, 27] and safety reports [28–30] indicate that cold medicines and opioids may represent risks of ADRs, particularly in younger children. As it is shown in **Table 4**, the majority of UMC reports are associated to diphenhydramine and dextromethorphan. Codeine reports are still growing.

Age/drug	DM	Guaifenesin	Pseudoe	PE	BH	CP	DH	Codeine
0–27 days	9	4	66	13	3	93	25	13
28 days to 23 months	149	103	217	76	13	287	274	136
2–11 years	825	194	502	79	21	703	741	429
12–17 years	600	95	471	37	8	356	604	277
Total	1583	396	1256	205	45	1439	1644	855

DM, dextromethorphan; GUA, guaifenesin; pseudo, pseudoephedrine; PE, phenylephrine; BH, brompheniramine; CP, chlorpheniramine; DH, diphenhydramine. Source: vigiaccess.org

Table 4.
Number of ADRs in children from UMC reports of some cold medicine.

5. A Latin American experience in ADR prospective study

5.1 Study design and participants

A prospective observational cohort study based on intensive pharmacovigilance was conducted from June to December 2013 in two general pediatric wards located in a city of the Colombian Caribbean Coast. One hospital was private and included 20 bed capacity units, from which isolation beds are assigned on a need basis. The other hospital was public with 29 bed capacity units, two of which are used for isolated patients. Both hospitals admit children between the neonatal period and 17 years of age.

This study included 1056 pediatric patients of ≤5 years of age (including neonates) without ADRs which were hospitalized at least 24 hours and had at least one prescribed medication. Researchers followed the patients until discharge. All parents authorized children participation and signed a consent. Patients were excluded if they were admitted only for taking diagnostic test or referred from other institutions. In addition, side effects associated with the administration of intravenous solutions, contrast media, nutraceuticals, and topical products were not monitored.

5.2 Data collection

Data collection was conducted by a clinical nurse who was trained in ADR detection. Daily visits to the wards were conducted. The instrument had two sections; the first one contained a sociodemographic variables, medical history, and information about previous medicines. The second one was an adaptation of the Yellow Card Scheme. All data from nursing, medical, and clinical laboratory test records were evaluated in order to detect suspected ADRs. A suspected ADR was defined as "any deviation of the expected clinical status (signs, symptoms and other clinical and laboratory findings)" [31].

The modified Schumock and Thornton criteria [32] were used to evaluate preventability. Naranjo's algorithm was employed to evaluate the temporal relationship and the biological/pharmacological plausibility between drug exposure and suspected ADR [33], while the severity was judged using modified Hartwig and Siegel Assessment Scale [34]. The team employed for analyzing the aspects was multidisciplinary (a pharmacist, a nurse, a pharmacologist, and a pediatrician).

5.3 Statistical analysis

A descriptive analysis of the variables was conducted. A crude bivariate relative risk (RR) and 95% confidence interval (CI) were estimated between the presence or absence of ADRs (dependent variable) and other variables. A chi-square test ($p < 0.05$) was also done between the dependent variable and the other one.

5.4 Incidence and characteristics of ADRs

Due to physiological and pharmacological differences between neonates and children of other ages, the results of this research are presented in a comparative way.

Two hundred seventy-nine ADRs were detected in 225 children. The cumulative incidence of ADRs was 21.31% (225/1056). Separately, neonate's incidence was 27.4% (78/284) and ≤5 years of age was 19.0% (147/772) [21, 22].

In neonates, 0.81% (1) of the ADRs were classified as definite (certain), 82.93% (102) probable, and 16.26% (20) possible. About 98.37% (121) were not preventable and 1.63% (2) preventable. About 9.75% (12) of the ADRs were severe, 31.71% (39) moderate, and 58.74% (72) mild.

On the other hand, in children ≤5 years of age, 0.64% (1) of the ADRs were classified as definite (certain), 98.08% (153) probable, and 1.28% (2) possible. About 98.72% (154) were not preventable and 1.28% (2) preventable. In terms of severity, 66.03% (103) of the ADRs were mild and 33.97% (53) moderate.

The comparison is shown in **Table 5**, in which it shows higher rates of severe ADRs in neonates. It may be related with the complex treatment established in neonatal intensive care unit (NICU).

The most affected organ system in neonates was the hematologic. In children ≤5 years of age, the most affected organ system was digestive. The entire list is detailed in **Table 6**. In all cases, ADR treatment was the responsibility of physicians.

The therapeutic group that most frequently produced ADRs was systemic antibiotics, in both groups, neonates and children. This information is detailed in **Table 7**. This is mainly due to the high use of this group of drugs in children.

5.5 Factors associated with ADRs

The mean gestational age in neonates with ADRs was 34.5 weeks compared with 37.0 ($p = 0.003$) who did not have. Additionally, preterm newborns were 2.30 more likely to have an ADR compare with term (95% CI 1.31–4.01, $p = 0.003$). The mean of days of hospitalization in neonates who had ADRs was 18.5, in comparison with 7.0. Having a hospital stay less than ≤8 days is related with the nonappearance of ADR (RR = 0.076, 95% CI 0.037–0.156, $p = 0.000$) [21].

The mean age of children ≤5 years of age that developed ADRs was similar between both groups, the ones who had ADRs and the ones did not showed any. However, ADR frequency was higher in children under 2 years of age (12.70%) than in children with 2 or more years of age (6.30%). Male patients were more likely to develop ADRs (RR = 1.66; 95% CI 1.22–2.25, $p = 0.001$) than female [22].

The mean length of hospitalization in children ≤5 years of age who had ADRs was higher (7.1 days ±5.2) than those who did not show ADRs (5.3 days ±2.6, $p = <0.001$) [22]. The mean of prescribed medicines in children with ADRs was

Characteristics	Neonatal age n = 284		Children ≤5 years of age n = 772	
	N	%	N	%
Imputability (Naranjo's algorithm)				
Definite (certain)	1	0.81	1	0.64
Probable	102	82.93	153	98.08
Possible	20	16.26	2	1.28
Severity (Hartwig and Siegel scale)				
Severe	12	9.75	0	0
Moderate	39	31.71	53	33.97
Mild	72	58.54	103	66.03
Preventability				
Preventable	2	1.63	2	1.28
Not preventable	121	98.37	154	98.72

Table 5.
Characteristics of ADRs in Colombian children.

Organic system affected	Neonatal age n = 284		Children ≤5 years of age n = 772	
	N	%	N	%
Hematologic	42	34.15	2	1.28
Digestive	41	33.33	100	64.1
Renal	12	9.76	4	2.56
Integumentary	6	4.88	19	12.19
Cardiovascular	3	2.44	21	13.46
Others	19	15.44	10	6.41
Total of ADR	123	100	156	100

Table 6.
Organic system affected in neonates and children with ADRs.

ATC code	Neonatal age n = 284		Children ≤5 years of age n = 772	
	N	%	N	%
Anti-infectives for systemic use	99	80.49	110	70.51
Respiratory system	9	7.31	25	16.03
Systemic hormonal preparations*	1	0.81	7	4.49
Nervous system	2	1.63	8	5.13
Cardiovascular system	3	2.44	1	0.64
Blood and blood-forming organs	2	1.63	1	0.64
Alimentary tract and metabolism	0	0	4	2.56
Others	7	5.69	0	0
Total	123	100	156	100

ATC, anatomical therapeutic chemical classification.
*Excluding sex hormones and insulins.

Table 7.
ADRs presented by children.

higher than those who did not show any (mean 5.0 ± 2.5 vs. 3.9 ± 2.4 drugs) (p = <0.001). Similarly, the number of prescribed systemic antibiotics in children with ADRs was also higher than in those who were not prescribed any (mean 2.0 ± 0.5 vs. 1.0 ± 0.5) (p = <0.001). The use of systemic antibiotics was correlated with a higher risk of ADRs (RR = 1.82 (95% CI 1.17–2.82, p = 0.005)) than those who did not use an antibiotic (**Table 4**). About 1.5% (12) of patients with ADRs reported previous ADRs [22].

6. Discussion

We followed a cohort of 1056 hospitalized patients, among neonates and children ≤5 years of age. We identified an ADR incidence of 21.3%, which is higher than Jimenez et al. [35]. These results demonstrate that children are particularly susceptible to ADRs. A Cuban Research which included patients under 18 years of age found that the age range most affected by ADRs was between 2 and 11 years of age [36]. But we only included patients ≤5 years of age. Children ages were divided as <2 years and ≥2 years of age, due to biological variability. Males were more often affected by ADRs than females, similar to the WHO ICSR database (VigiBase ®), in which ADRs were primarily presented in males [18]. However, other studies have revealed higher ADRs rate in females [36, 37].

The mean of days of hospitalization in neonates who had ADRs was 18.5, in comparison with 7.0. The average length of hospitalization in older children was 7.1 days. This difference might be due to differences in neonates and children patients. The mean number of prescribed medicines in children with ADRs was similar to European and non-European countries who have reported an average number higher than 5 [33].

Respiratory drugs and systemic antibiotics were the therapeutic groups mostly associated with ADR incidence in both neonates and children. As noted, respiratory drugs and systemic antibiotics are not only the most prescribed class of drugs for hospitalized children but also the ones that usually cause ADRs. The most commons ADRs linked to systemic antibiotics were digestive for older children, while hemato-logic were for neonates. Similar findings were reported by Belen-Rivas et al. [19].

Most of the ADRs found in our study were mild. These results differ with the findings of Shamna et al. [39], who found that moderate ADRs were the most common. According with Naranjo's algorithm, the majority of ADRs were classified as probable; also Belen-Rivas [19] reported that the majority of ADRs were prob-able. The evaluation of ADRs is predisposed by the definitions, the methodology of detection, classification, and the study setting included.

The main limitation of this study was the determination of imputability of adverse events. Regardless of patient daily visits, only 0.81% of neonates and 0.64% of older children were categorized as definite ADRs. Naranjo's algorithm determines an ADR as definite when the drug is readministered or a placebo is administered and the drug serum level lab tests are carried out. In most cases, for ethical reasons, these are not feasible. Likewise, if a suspected ADR is detected, in most of the cases, the drug is ceased, which limits the ability to evaluate all the criteria for imput-ability. This study was purely observational, and no intervention was conducted on patient's treatment.

Even though we did not estimate a sample size due to difficulties in establishing the general population, an observation period of 6 months permitted us to measure an ADR incidence.

7. Conclusion

ADRs are common among inpatient neonates and children. In neonates, hav-ing less than ≤8 days of hospitalization is linked with the nonappearance of ADRs (RR = 0.076, 95% CI 0.037–0.156, p = 0.000). In children, males are more likely to develop ADRs (RR = 1.66; 95% CI 1.22–2.25, p = 0.001) than females. Even when in neonates, it is not a significant RR; males have higher rates of occurrence than females. Systemic antibiotics are correlated with a higher risk of ADRs (RR = 1.82 (95% CI 1.17–2.82, p = 0.005) in children. All these findings mean that ADR repre-sents an additional burden of morbidity and risk for pediatric patients, particularly in those who used several medicines.

Pharmacovigilance in pediatric population needs to be reinforced. It is necessary to develop a proactive pharmacovigilance and patient safety programs with a focus in risk analysis and management, in which ADR reporting should be mandatory. This measure might help us make our health-care systems safer, especially for children, in which this topic must be further investigated.

For succeeding in ADR detection, it is important to have a team conformed by physicians, nurses, pharmacists, and others (according to the health service). In addition, it should be noted that, due to the role nurses play in the administration and monitoring of therapy, they have a privileged position to detect drug effects, including ADRs.

In order to prevent ADRs, it is advisable to generate strategies that are aimed at improving drug administration safety protocols.

Acknowledgements

Authors thank Colciencias for funding the project related to ADRs in Colombian children. We are grateful with the hospitals, the nurses, the pediatricians, and the pharmacist who collaborated during data collection and analysis. This project was supported by Grant 566–2012. Also, authors thank "Universidad del Norte" (Barranquilla, Colombia) and the Department of Nursing for giving us the time to develop this chapter. Thanks to Daniela Díaz for the data collection and analysis.

Conflict of interest

The authors declare no conflict of interest.

Ethical considerations

The protocol was approved by the Research Ethics Committee of the Health Care Division of the "Universidad del Norte" and was declared as minimal risk by the researchers. Likewise, the protocol was conducted under the human research ethical criteria defined as the Declaration of Helsinki.

Appendices and nomenclature

ADR	adverse drug reaction
OTC	over the counter
WHO	World Health Organization
NICU	neonatal intensive care unit
UMC	Uppsala Monitoring Centre
NSAIDs	non-steroidal anti-inflammatories

Author details

Roxana De Las Salas[1*] and Claudia Margarita Vásquez Soto[2]

1 Universidad del Norte, Barranquilla, Colombia

2 Hospital Universidad del Norte, Barranquilla, Colombia

*Address all correspondence to: rdelassalas@uninorte.edu.co

IntechOpen

References

[1] World Health Organization. The importance of pharmacovigilance. Safety Monitoring of Medicinal Product. United Kingdom: World Health Organization; 2002. Available from: http://apps.who.int/medicinedocs/pdf/s4893e/s4893e.pdf?ua=1 [Accessed: 2018-06-30]

[2] Caron J, Rochoy M, Gaboriau L, Gautier S. The history of pharmacovigilance. Therapie. 2016;71(2):129-134

[3] Wax PM. Elixirs, diluents, and the passage of the 1938 Federal Food, Drug and Cosmetic Act. Annals of Internal Medicine. 1995;122(6):456-461

[4] The Uppsala Monitoring Centre. Glossary of terms used in Pharmacovigilance. Uppsala: UMC, 2011. Available from: http://who-umc.org/Graphics/24729.pdf [Accessed: 2018-06-20]

[5] AEMPS. Information for Notifications of Suspected Adverse Drug Reactions by Health Professionals. Spain: AEMPS; 2015. Available from: https://www.aemps.gob.es/vigilancia/medicamentosUsoHumano/SEFV-H/NRA-SEFV-H/notificaSospechas-RAM-profSanitarios.htm [Accessed: 2018-06-30]

[6] Lu H, Rosenbaum S. Developmental pharmacokinetics in pediatric populations. The Journal of Pediatric Pharmacology and Therapeutics. 2014;19(4):262-276

[7] O'Hara K, Wright IMR, Schneider JJ, Jones AL, Martin JH. Pharmacokinetics in neonatal prescribing: Evidence base, paradigms and the future. British Journal of Clinical Pharmacology. 2015;80(6):1281-1288

[8] Hennessy S, Strom BL. PDUFA reauthorization—Drug safety's golden moment of opportunity? New England Journal of Medicine. 2007;356:1703-1704

[9] Vallano A, Cereza G, Pedrós C, Agustí A, Danés I, Aguilera C, et al. Obstacles and solutions for spontaneous reporting of adverse drug reactions in the hospital. British Journal of Clinical Pharmacology. 2005;60(6):653-658

[10] Raine J. Pharmacovigilance in Paediatric Population. The PRAC's perspective EU: EMA; 2014

[11] Thiesen S, Conroy EJ, Bellis JR, Bracken LE, Mannix HL, Bird KA, et al. Incidence, characteristics and risk factors of adverse drug reactions in hospitalized children—A prospective observational cohort study of 6,601 admissions. BMC Medicine. 2013;11(1):1-10

[12] Temple ME, Robinson RF, Miller JC, Hayes JR, Nahata MC. Frequency and preventability of adverse drug reactions in paediatric patients. Drug Safety. 2004;27(11):819-829

[13] Pan American Health Organization. Good pharmacovigilance practices for the Americas. PANDRH Technical Document N° 5. Washington, DC: PAHO; 2011. Available from: http://apps.who.int/medicinedocs/documents/s18625en/s18625en.pdf Accessed: 2018-06-30

[14] Turner MA, Hill H. Pharmacovigilance in neonatal intensive care. In: Mimouni F, van den Anker JN, editors. Neonatal Pharmacology and Nutrition Update. 18. Basel: Karger; 2015. pp. 28-40

[15] Du W, Lehr VT, Lieh-Lai M, Koo W, Ward RM, Rieder MJ, et al. An algorithm to detect adverse drug reactions in the neonatal intensive care

unit. Journal of Clinical Pharmacology. 2013;**53**(1):87-95

[16] Healthcare Ministry. Improving Patient Safety in Medicines Use. Colombia: Healthcare Ministry; 2010. Available from: https://www.minsalud. gov.co/sites/rid/Lists/BibliotecaDigital/ RIDE/DE/CA/seguridad-en-la-utilizacion-de-medicamentos.pdf [Accessed: 2018-06-30]

[17] Sharma B, Bhattacharya A, Gandhi R, Sood J, Rao B. Pharmacovigilance in intensive care unit—An overview. Indian Journal of Anaesthesia. 2008;**52**:373

[18] Star K, Noren GN, Nordin K, Edwards IR. Suspected adverse drug reactions reported for children worldwide: an exploratory study using VigiBase. Drug Safety. 2011;**34**(5):415-428

[19] Belén-Rivas A, Arruza L, Pacheco E, Portoles A, Diz J, Vargas E. Adverse drug reactions in neonates: A prospective study. Archives of Disease in Childhood. 2016;**101**(4):371-376

[20] Vázquez-Alvarez AO, Brennan-Bourdon LM, Rincón-Sánchez AR, Islas-Carbajal MC, Huerta-Olvera SG. Improved drug safety through intensive pharmacovigilance in hospitalized pediatric patients. BMC Pharmacology & Toxicology. 2017;**18**:79

[21] De las Salas R, Díaz-Agudelo D. Reacciones adversas a medicamentos en neonatos hospitalizados en unidades de cuidado intensivo neonatal en Barranquilla, Colombia. Biomédica. 2017;**37**:33-42

[22] De las salas R, Díaz-Agudelo D, Burgos-Flórez FJ, Vaca C, Serrano-Meriño DV. Adverse drug reactions in hospitalized colombian children. Colombia Médica. 2016;**47**(3):2016

[23] dos Santos DB, Coelho HL. Adverse drug reactions in hospitalized children in Fortaleza, Brazil. Pharmacoepidemiology and Drug Safety. 2006;**15**(9):635-640

[24] Sharek PJ, Horbar JD, Mason W, Bisarya H, Thurm CW, Suresh G, et al. Adverse events in the neonatal intensive care unit: development, testing, and findings of an NICU-focused trigger tool to identify harm in North American NICUs. Pediatrics. 2006;**118**(4):1332-1340

[25] Digra KK, Pandita A, Saini GS, Bharti R. Pattern of adverse drug reactions in children attending the department of pediatrics in a tertiary care center: A prospective observational study. Clinical Medicine Insights Pediatrics. 2015;**9**:73-78

[26] Paul IM, Reynolds KM, Green JL. Adverse events associated with opioid-containing cough and cold medications in children. Clinical Toxicology (Phila). 2018:1-3

[27] Etminan M, Nouri MR, Sodhi M, Carleton BC. Dentists' prescribing of analgesics for children in British Columbia. Canada. Journal of the Canadian Dental Association. 2017;**83**:h5

[28] FDA. FDA Drug Safety Communication: FDA Requires Labeling Changes for Prescription Opioid Cough and Cold Medicines to Limit their Use to Adults 18 Years and Older. USA: FDA; 2018. Available from: https://www.fda.gov/Safety/ MedWatch/SafetyInformation/ SafetyAlertsforHumanMedical Products/ucm590435.htm [Accessed: 2018-06-30]

[29] FDA. FDA Drug Safety Communication: FDA Restricts Use of Prescription Codeine Pain and Cough Medicines and Tramadol Pain Medicines in Children; Recommends Against Use

in Breastfeeding Women. USA: FDA; 2017. Available from: https://www.fda.gov/Drugs/DrugSafety/ucm549679.htm [Accessed: 2018-06-30]

[30] FDA. FDA Drug Safety Communication: FDA Evaluating the Potential Risks of Using Codeine Cough-and-Cold Medicines in Children. USA: FDA; 2015. https://www.fda.gov/Drugs/DrugSafety/ucm453125.htm. Available from: [Accessed: 2018-06-30]

[31] International Conference on Harmonisation (ICH). Post-approval Safety Data Management: Definitions and Standards for Expedited Reporting E2D; 2003. http://www.ich.org/fileadmin/Public_Web_Site/ICH_Products/Guidelines/Efficacy/E2D/Step4/E2D_Guideline.pdf [Accessed: 2018-04-30]

[32] Schumock GT, Thornton JP. Focusing on the preventability of adverse drug reactions. Hospital Pharmacy. 1992;**27**(6):538

[33] Naranjo C, Busto U, Sellers E, Sandor P, Ruiz I, Roberts E, et al. A method for estimating the probability of adverse drug reactions. Clinical Pharmacology & Therapeutics. 1981;**30**(2):239-245

[34] Hartwig SC, Siegel J, Schneider PJ. Preventability and severity assessment in reporting adverse drug reactions. American Journal of Hospital Pharmacy. 1992;**49**(9):2229-2232

[35] Jimenez R, Smith A, Carleton B. New ways of detecting ADRs in neonates and children. Current Pharmaceutical Design. 2015;**21**(39):5643-5649

[36] Furones Mourelle JA, Cruz Barrios MA, López Aguilera ÁF, Martínez Núñez D, Alfonso Orta I. Reacciones adversas por antimicrobianos en niños de Cuba. Revista Cubana de Medicina General Integral. 2015;**31**(2):205-216

[37] Li H, Guo X-J, Ye X-F, Jiang H, Du W-M, Xu J-F, et al. Adverse drug reactions of spontaneous reports in Shanghai pediatric population. PLoS One. 2014;**9**(2):e89829

[38] Rashed A, Wong IK, Cranswick N, Tomlin S, Rascher W, Neubert A. Risk factors associated with adverse drug reactions in hospitalised children: International multicentre study. European Journal of Clinical Pharmacology. 2012;**68**(5):801-810

[39] Shamna M, Dilip C, Ajmal M, Linu Mohan P, Shinu C, Jafer CP, et al. A prospective study on adverse drug reactions of antibiotics in a tertiary care hospital. Saudi Pharmaceutical Journal. 2014;**22**(4):303-338

Active Pharmacovigilance in Epileptic Patients: A Deep Insight into Phenytoin Behaviour

Marta Vázquez, Pietro Fagiolino, Cecilia Maldonado,
Natalia Guevara, Manuel Ibarra, Isabel Rega,
Adriana Gómez, Antonella Carozzi and Carlos Azambuja

Abstract

Despite the introduction of new and more expensive anticonvulsant drugs, phenytoin (PHT) is still a first-line medication for common types of epilepsy such as tonic-clonic and complex partial seizures but not for absence seizures. PHT shows a nonlinear kinetics and a narrow therapeutic range, thus a fine balance must be found between efficacy and toxic effects. Since the free (unbound) drug is responsible for producing the pharmacological effect, the concentration in a novel biological fluid more closely related to arterial free plasma drug concentration—saliva—is used in this study as part of the monitoring strategy. Therefore, in order to optimize therapy in epileptic patients under PHT treatment, plasma and saliva concentrations of PHT were measured, and adverse drug reactions were registered during a 2-year follow-up. CYP2C9, CYP2C19, and epoxide hydrolase polymorphisms (enzymes involved in PHT metabolism) were also analyzed using, in this way, pharmacogenetics for drug safety. The two PHT brands commercially available in our country and used in this study demonstrated similar pattern of efficacy and safety.

Keywords: phenytoin, pharmacovigilance, therapeutic drug monitoring, pharmacokinetics, pharmacogenetics

1. Introduction

Phenytoin (PHT) is approved to be used for almost any type of epilepsy such as generalized tonic-clonic and complex partial (psychomotor and temporal lobe) seizures and for preventing and treating seizures occurring during or following neurosurgery except for absence seizures [1]. Regarding its mechanism of action, PHT exerts a stabilizing effect on excitable membranes of several cells, including neurons and cardiac myocytes. It inhibits voltage-dependent sodium channels, reducing sodium flow during action potential [2]. Taking into account, PHT has a narrow therapeutic range; therapies with this drug are monitored by plasma quantification in the routine practice [3]. However, when using plasma drug concentrations in therapeutic drug monitoring (TDM), free plus protein bound drug is measured. As it is known, plasma or serum concentration does not usually represent the concentration at its receptor site. Only free drug can reach the biophase (action site) and interact with a receptor to produce the effect (therapeutic or toxic). Total drug concentrations depend on protein binding, and PHT is highly bound to albumin. But, free drug monitoring is rather expensive for routine practice. Our research group has been working for several years using saliva as biological fluid [4–6]. Saliva is not only useful for being a simple and noninvasive collection method but also for the information it gives. Studies have demonstrated that salivary concentrations highly correlate with free drug concentration in plasma mainly for drugs, which are lipophilic and nonionized at salivary pH (i.e., phenytoin or carbamazepine), and therefore, saliva concentrations are more reflective of the concentration at the biophase. Saliva is produced in the salivary glands by ultrafiltration of arterial plasma. Arterial drug concentration is higher than the respective venous concentration during drug input either after intravenous or oral administration [7]. So if enterohepatic or blood-gastrointestinal cycling processes are operating, elevated saliva drug concentrations (reflecting higher arterial drug concentrations) during the elimination phase could predict re-entry processes. Using this fluid, our research group has studied enterohepatic recirculation of paracetamol [8] and blood gastrointestinal cycling of methadone [9].

It is important to note that for the treatment of epilepsy, the effective and safe plasma concentrations referenced in the literature are between 10 and 20 mg/L, and salivary concentrations are between 1 and 2 mg/L. The narrow population therapeutic range, the clinical consequences of presenting subtherapeutic or toxic concentrations, and the difficulty of determining the pharmacokinetic parameters for each patient predispose the clinician to follow the therapy with this anticonvulsant agent through a frequent determination of plasma and/or salivary concentrations in each patient. Therefore, the dose range compatible with a therapeutic serum or a saliva concentration is narrow within subjects, and TDM is of particular value in dosage tailoring [3, 10].

PHT is a weak acid, which usually administered as the sodium salt. Its solubility in water is scarce even in the intestine as it precipitates at the intestinal pH, a fact that conditions its entry into the body. However, it is well absorbed when administered orally, with a bioavailability close to 90%, which implies that in addition to the great lipophilicity that it presents, the metabolism at the enterocyte level is low. The drug has a volume of distribution of 0.64 L/kg and is approximately 90% bound to plasma proteins [10, 11]. PHT main biotransformation route is para-hydroxylation to form the inactive metabolite 5-(4-hydroxyphenyl)-5-phenylhydantoin (p-HPPH). The enzyme involved in this step is CYP2C9 and, to a lesser extent, CYP2C19 [11]. p-HPPH formation occurs via an arene-oxide intermediate, and the accumulation of the latter can be the cause of skin reactions associated with PHT [12, 13]. Further oxidation of p-HPPH leads to catechol formation (3'-4'-diHPPH), by CYP2C9, CYP2C19, and CYP3A4, also undergoing an arene-oxide intermediate. On the other side, the arene oxide can also be converted to transdihydrodiol phenytoin via microsomal epoxide hydrolase (EPXH), which can also lead to catechol formation. The enzymes CYP2C9, CYP2C19, and EPHX are polymorphically expressed [14–16].

There is strong evidence that PHT undergoes an important secretion from blood to the digestive tract after which the drug would re-enter the body from the intestinal lumen. Observations of secondary peaks in plasma concentration profiles after intravenous doses of PHT constitute strong arguments to affirm the important contribution of recirculation between internal medium and gastrointestinal lumen in the pharmacokinetics of this drug [17–19].

PHT was traditionally believed to saturate the hepatic enzymes and thereafter giving rise to a nonlinear concentration-dose relationship, described by the Michaelis-Menten equation. An alternative hypothesis based on its ability to induce efflux transporters was reported by our group, and this inductive effect was demonstrated in rats to be time-and-concentration-dependent [20–22]. The efflux transporter involved would be MRP2, and by means of this efflux pump, the drug would be secreted, in an important way, towards the digestive tract, thus propitiating the appearance of secondary peaks even after its intravenous administration. The induction of its expression would slow the oral absorption of PHT, a fact that is noticeable when analyzing the plasma profiles of the drug during the interval of administration in multiple doses, which are much less acute than the profiles observed after single doses. On the other hand, the deviation of the drug from the liver to the intestine would avoid the major biotransformation that takes place in the hepatocyte. Given the greater abundance of CYP2C9 and CYP2C19 enzymes present in the liver in relation to the enterocytes, a reduction in clearance in a concentration-dependent manner as verified during chronic treatments could be observed. In other words, the nonlinear kinetics found for this drug would not correspond to an enzymatic saturation but to an induction in the expression of transporters that remove molecules from the sites of high metabolism [20, 22].

The toxic effects of PHT depend on the route of administration, the duration of exposure, and the dose [23]. When administered IV with an excessive speed for status epilepticus, the most important toxic signs are cardiac arrhythmias with or without hypotension and central nervous system depression. These complications are reduced with the slow administration of diluted solutions of the drug. IV administration of PHT should not exceed 50 mg/minute for adults and should be well diluted in physiological solution in order to reduce local venous irritation due to the alkalinity of drug solutions [24–26].

The toxic effects associated with chronic treatment include concentration-related effects, as well as confusion, behavioral disturbances, increased frequency of seizures, gastrointestinal symptoms, hirsutism, gingival hyperplasia, osteomalacia, and megaloblastic anemia. Undesirable effects include vertigo, ataxia, headache, diplopia, and nystagmus but not sedation. Increased incidence of fetal malformations (mainly cleft palate) has been observed in children born from epileptic mothers under PHT treatment. Occasionally, increased hepatic transaminases are also observed [27].

The reported endocrine effects are diverse. Osteomalacia with hypocalcemia and increased alkaline phosphatase has been attributed both to an increased vitamin D metabolism due to the inducing effect of PHT and to inhibition of intestinal calcium absorption. PHT also increases the metabolism of vitamin K and reduces the concentration of vitamin K-dependent proteins that are important for the normal metabolism of calcium in bone [28].

Hypersensitivity reactions can vary from mild rashes in 2–5% of patients to sometimes more severe and life-threatening skin reactions such as Stevens-Johnson syndrome [29].

Active pharmacovigilance, in contrast to passive, seeks to ascertain the number of adverse reactions (lack of efficacy or toxicity) via a continuous process. An example of active surveillance is the follow-up of patients treated with a particular drug. In general, it is more feasible to get more comprehensive data from the particular drug behavior through an active pharmacovigilance system than through a passive reporting system.

Nowadays, two commercial brands of PHT are available in Uruguay for oral administration, both multisource drug products (Antepil® and Comitoína®). Due to the characteristics of PHT previously mentioned, there is a need to evaluate these products in their natural clinical setting because the clinical response is never assessed in bioequivalence studies carried out with healthy volunteers.

2. Objective

The objective of this study was to optimize PHT therapeutics by active pharmacovigilance in epileptic patients under PHT treatment (either Antepil® or Comitoína®) measuring plasma and saliva concentrations, determining CYP2C9, CYP2C19, and epoxide hydrolase (EPHX) polymorphisms, registering adverse drug reactions (ADR) during a 2-year time period, and demonstrating that both PHT brands have similar pattern of efficacy and safety.

3. Patients and methods

3.1 Subjects and design

The inclusion criteria for patients included a diagnosis of epilepsy carried out by the attending neurologist. Some patients were treated only with Antepil® for the study period of 2 years, and some were treated only with Comitoína® during the same period. Patients with hepatic or renal impairment, pregnant and lactating women, and individuals with history of alcohol or drug abuse or addiction or with diminished intellectual or motor abilities were excluded from the study. The study protocol was approved by the Institutional Ethics Review Committee of the Faculty of Chemistry, Universidad de la República, and written consent was obtained from all subjects prior to their participation in the study.

All the information about PHT concentrations in plasma and saliva, PHT dose and dosing interval, comedications, adverse effects (lack of efficacy or toxic effects), and laboratories results (liver and renal function and hemogram tests, albumin in blood) of the patients were collected by the pharmacists of the program using a data sheet elaborated for this purpose every time the patient came for the interview and for blood and saliva analysis (see Section 3.2).

One electroencephalogram in the 2-year period was also obtained.

Patients also had a form in which they wrote down any ADR they experienced, indicating start time and duration. Patients called the neurologists of the pharmacovigilance program when an ADR occurred and the physician determined the action to take and communicated this action to the pharmacists. All the ADRs were notified to the Pharmacovigilance Unit of the Health Ministry completing the Yellow Form. The causality assessment of ADRs was carried out using Naranjo's algorithm as shown in **Table 1**.

3.2 Sampling and chemical analysis

The pharmacovigilance protocol includes predose blood and saliva samples every 3 months and salivary curves when the subject was included in the study and 1 year later. Laboratory tests were performed twice in the 2-year period except for albumin in blood that was carried out in every occasion.

Predose blood samples (5 mL) were taken from the antecubital vein and placed into heparinized tubes, and saliva samples were obtained by stimulation with citric acid and scheduled before dose intake and at 1, 2, 3, 4, 5, 6, 8, and 12 hours after dosing. Blood and saliva samples were centrifuged and stored in freezer ($-25°C$) until analysis.

Quantification of PHT in saliva was carried out by Chemiluminescent Microparticle Immunoassay (CMIA), using Architect (Abbot™) equipment, according to the instructions given in the package insert. Precision and accuracy were below

Question	Yes	No	Do not know	Score
1. Are there previous conclusive reports on this reaction?	+1	0	0	
2. Did the adverse event appear after the suspected drug was administered?	+2	−1	0	
3. Did the adverse event improve when the drug was discontinued or a specific antagonist was administered?	+1	0	0	
4. Did the adverse event reappear when the drug was readministered?	+2	−1	0	
5. Are there alternative causes that could on their own have caused the reaction?	−1	+2	0	
6. Did the reaction reappear when a placebo was given?	−1	+1	0	
7. Was the drug detected in blood or other fluids in concentrations known to be toxic?	+1	0	0	
8. Was the reaction more severe when the dose was increased or less severe when the dose was decreased?	+1	0	0	
9. Did the patient have a similar reaction to the same or similar drugs in any previous exposure?	+1	0	0	
10. Was the adverse event confirmed by any objective evidence?	+1	0	0	
			Total score:	

Total score: >9 = definitive reaction, 5–8 = probable, 1–4 = possible, ≤0 = doubtful.

Table 1.
Naranjo's casuality algorithm.

15% and between 85 and 115%, respectively, except at the lower limit of quantification (0.3 mg/L), where intra- and inter-day coefficient of variation rose up to 20%.

Plasma PHT and p-HPHH concentrations were determined by a high performance liquid chromatography (HPLC) method based on a procedure previously published by Savio et al. [30]. The method was linear between 0.5286 mg/L (the lower limit of quantification, LLOQ) and 24.39 mg/L for PHT and between 0.0585 mg/L (LLOQ) and 2.701 mg/L for p-HPPH.

3.3 Pharmacokinetic and statistical analysis

The following pharmacokinetic parameters at steady state (ss) were determined from the experimental salivary PHT concentration curves versus time:

- Area under the saliva PHT concentration-time curve from 0 to T hours (AUCss $0–T$) calculated by the linear trapezoidal rule with T being the administration interval.

- Experimental maximum and minimum concentration (Cmaxss and Cminss) of the curve.

- Time to obtain maximum concentration (Tmaxss).

- Mean concentration (Cmeanss = AUCss $0–T/T$).

- Peak-to-trough fluctuation [PTF = (Cmaxss − Cminss) × 100/Cmeanss].

The statistical processing of the information was carried out using the statistical program Statistical Package for the Social Sciences, version 17 (SPSS), and it was by obtaining mean values, standard deviations, and 95% confidence intervals (95% CI) of the pharmacokinetic parameters.

3.4 Genotyping procedure of EPHX, CYP2C9, and CYP2C19

Genotyping procedure of EPHX, CYP2C9, and CYP2C19 was carried out by Genia (Molecular Genetics Laboratory, Montevideo, Uruguay). EPHX polymorphism was done by real-time polymerase chain reaction (RT-PCR). To determine CYP2C9 and 2C19 genotype, a conventional PCR was performed for each SNP (rs 1799853 and rs 1057910 for CYP2C9; rs 4244285 and rs 4986893 for CYP2C19). The complete technique is specified in the study performed by our group [31].

3.5 *In vitro* dissolution study

Six units of each product were tested in Distek® Dissolution System 2100C equipment. The conditions were as follows: USP 32 Apparatus 2 (paddle); 75 rpm stirring speed; volume 900 mL of water; and temperature 37 ± 0.5°C. Samples were automatically withdrawn by the use of an Agilent 89092EO pump at 10, 15, 20, 30, 40, 60, and 80 minutes. The drug release at different time intervals was measured by UV-visible spectrophotometer (Agilent 8453 and ChemStation® software).

4. Results and discussion

A total of 57 adult Caucasian epileptic subjects were included in the active pharmacovigilance program. Thirty-three individuals were receiving a conventional dose of Antepil® 100 mg (Fármaco Uruguayo Laboratory) and 24 of Comitoína® 100 mg (Roemmers Laboratory). The demographic characteristics of the subjects for Antepil® and Comitoína® are summarized in **Tables 2** and **3**, respectively.

The *in vitro* dissolution assay demonstrated a slow release drug rate for both brands as it can be seen in **Figure 1** but with a faster onset for Antepil®. This is in accordance with the saliva concentration-time profiles of both brands as shown in **Figures 2** and **3**. Although the saliva profiles are similar, a delay at the beginning of the absorption can be seen in Comitoína® profile (**Figure 3**).

Several secondary peaks can be observed after diurnal administration of PHT (**Figures 2** and **3**), and this is evidencing the PHT recirculation processes that have already been studied by our group and other researchers as it was stated in Section 1. PHT could be stored in the digestive system organs to be later excreted to the small intestine lumen, from where it can re-enter into the bloodstream. This phenomenon would be favored by the overexpression of efflux transporters at the bile canaliculus caused by PHT, which would accelerate the escape of PHT molecules from hepatocyte that is the main site of drug metabolism by CYP2C9 and CYP2C19,

	Total	Male	Female
Subjects	33	15	18
Age (years)	46.6 (18–75)	42.0 (18–73)	50.4 (20–75)
Weight (kg)	75.8 (45–140)	75.9 (49–140)	75.7 (45–120)

Table 2.
Demographic characteristics of the patients under Antepil® treatment expressed as mean (95% CI).

deviating it to the intestinal lumen where metabolizing enzyme expression is poor, an adverse from where it would be available to re-entry into the bloodstream. As it can be observed in both figures, there is no important PTF.

Mean plasma protein binding of PHT was 89% for Antepil® and 90% for Comitoína®, which do not differ from the literature (80–90%). The plasma protein binding (PPB) was obtained as follows:

$$PPB = 100 \times (1 - [So]/[Po]). \qquad (1)$$

Being So and Po predose saliva and plasma concentration, respectively.

	Total	Male	Female
Subjects	24	12	12
Age (years)	45.8 (18–76)	47.8 (25–76)	44.0 (18–69)
Weight (kg)	76.5 (48–108)	80.1 (54–100)	66.9 (48–108)

Table 3.
Demographic characteristics of the patients under Comitoína® treatment expressed as mean (95% CI).

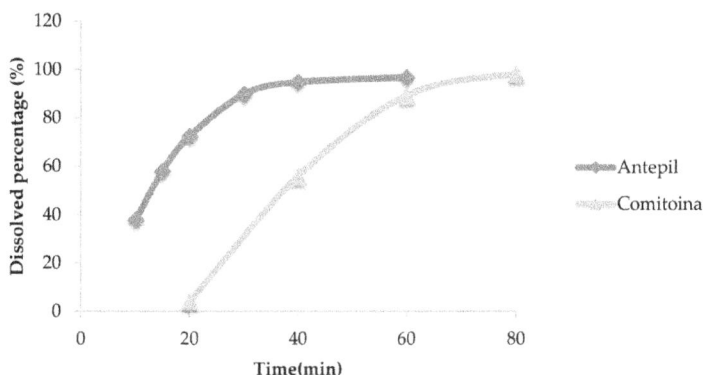

Figure 1.
Dissolution profile of the two brands of phenytoin in water.

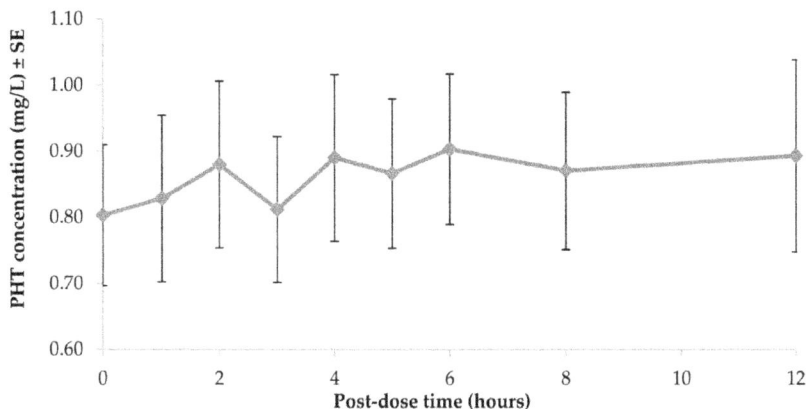

Figure 2.
Mean (±standard error) saliva PHT concentration-time profile after the administration of Antepil®.

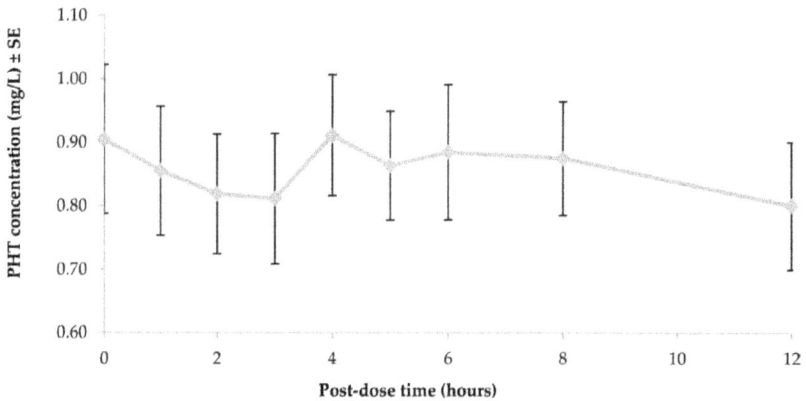

Figure 3.
Mean (±standard error) saliva PHT concentration-time profile after the administration of Comitoína®.

Serum albumin levels were between the reference range (3.30–5.00 g/dL) in all the subjects and in every occasion. No laboratories abnormalities were observed for any subject or brand during the 2-year study, except for ammonia levels determined only in some patients comedicated with valproic acid (VPA).

No significant differences were found in the normalized doses or in the salivary and plasma concentrations between men and women for either brand. However, there is a tendency for women to have lower plasma and saliva PHT concentration for equal normalized doses. Further studies with a greater number of individuals are needed to confirm this tendency. The explanation could be a greater apparent clearance in women due to either a higher systemic clearance of the drug or a lower oral bioavailability. Both could be probably given the greater expression of MRP2 and the higher fraction of cardiac output delivered to the intestine that women present in comparison to men.

Figures 4 and **5** show both plasma and salivary drug concentrations in response to the administered daily doses for Comitoína® and Antepil®, respectively.

Both **Figures 4** and **5** show the typical curvature of Michaelis-Menten kinetics described in the literature for plasma concentrations, considering a limited enzyme capacity. However, as explained in Section 1, an alternative hypothesis could explain the nonlinear kinetics of PHT. The decrease in clearance observed with increasing concentrations would be secondary to the induction of drug secretion from the blood into the intestine, from where it is subsequently reabsorbed. A concentration-local induction dependent on the transport of efflux caused by PHT itself would enhance the processes that prolong its permanence in the splanchnic zone. This would lead to a decrease in the amount of drug metabolized in the liver and a greater percentage of it would enter the process of enterohepatic recirculation, sending the drug to an area of poor metabolism such as the intestine from which it enters the body again. This effect could be responsible for both the low peak-to-trough fluctuation mentioned earlier and the disproportionate increase in plasma concentrations with dose increase.

The most common antiepileptic comedications in the patients included in the study were carbamazepine, lamotrigine, levetiracetam, and valproic acid.

Most adverse reactions with both Antepil® and Comitoína® did not deserve dose reduction according to the neurologist due to the fact that they were related to chronic treatment with PHT. The exception was the appearance of seizures with high PHT concentrations, which was considered as a possible concentration-dependent adverse reaction. PHT concentrations are responsible for the overexpression of

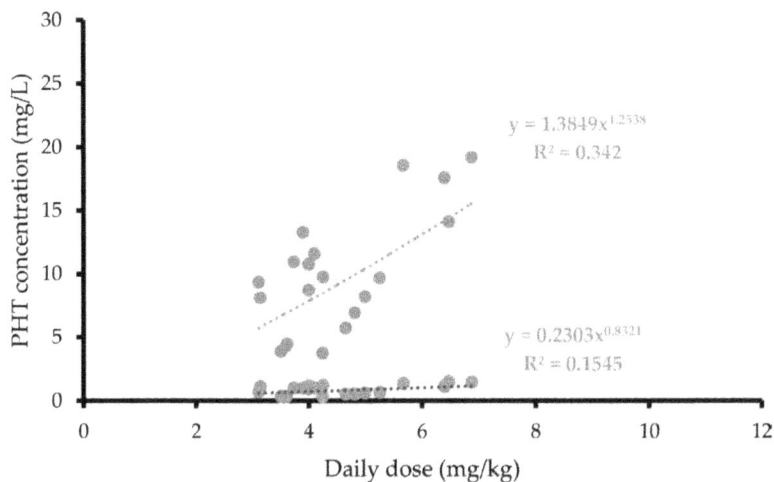

Figure 4.
Relationship between the normalized dose of PHT and plasma concentration (in red) and salivary concentration (in blue) for Comitoína®.

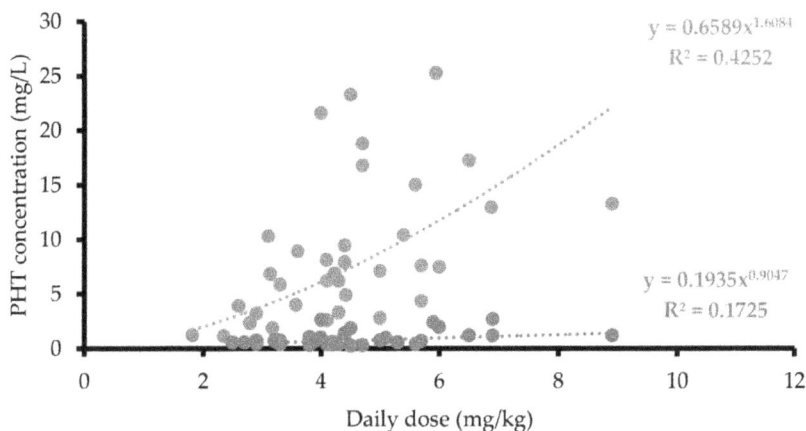

Figure 5.
Relationship between the normalized dose of PHT and plasma concentration (in red) and salivary concentration (in blue) for Antepil®.

efflux transporters, not only in the splanchnic zone but also in the hematoencephalic barrier, which could be the reason for low PHT levels in the brain and the appearance of seizures.

Some patients taking Antepil® were comedicated with VPA. Ammonia levels in some of these patients were higher than the upper limit of the normal range in blood (25–94 μg/dL). Our research group has been studying increased ammonia levels in patients under VPA treatment [32, 33]. High levels of ammonia in the brain can be the cause of seizures as ammonia easily crosses the blood-brain barrier, and in the brain, it can conjugate with α-ketoglutarate to form glutamate. This leads to brain damage and the appearance of seizures given the excitatory activity of glutamate in the synaptic membrane.

Tables 4 and **5** show the detected ADRs in patients under Antepil® or Comitoína® treatment, respectively, and the causality assessment using Naranjo's algorithm.

ADRs	Causality		Total
	Possible	Probable	
Gastrointestinal disorders	1	3	4
Visual problems	0	3	3
Drowsiness	3	0	3
Dizziness	2	1	3
Dysarthria	0	3	3
Bleeding gums/hyperplasia	0	1	1
Memory loss	0	1	1
Tremor in hands	0	1	1
Trouble in sleeping	0	2	2
Lack of strength in lower limbs	2	0	2
Orthostatic hypotension	0	1	1
Walk instability	1	1	2
Seizures*	1	3	4
Total	10	20	30

Seizures were reported as toxic reactions and not treatment failure when plasma levels of PHT were greater than 20 mg/L and when once the dose was reduced seizures disappear. In one patient, this adverse effect was assessed as possible as the patient was comedicated with VPA (1200 mg) and the ammonia level was 165.8 µg/dL, and as it was explained previously, VPA provoking hyperammonemia could be the cause of the seizures. Predose plasma levels of PHT and VPA were 24.8 and 49.7 mg/L, respectively, in this patient.

Table 4.
Detected adverse drug reactions (ADRs) and causality assessment in patients under Antepil® treatment.

ADRs	Causality		Total
	Possible	Probable	
Gastrointestinal disorders	2	1	3
Visual problems	3	5	8
Drowsiness	0	7	7
Dizziness	1	5	6
Dysarthria	1	2	3
Bleeding gums/hyperplasia	0	7	7
Memory loss	0	4	4
Walk instability	0	1	1
Tremor in hands	1	0	1
Headaches	0	1	1
Belly swelling	1	0	1
Irritability	0	1	1
Nervousness	0	1	1
Total	9	35	44

Table 5.
Detected adverse drug reactions (ADRs) and causality assessment in patients under Comitoína® treatment.

None of the patients developed skin reactions, an adverse effect observed in a clinical trial with healthy volunteers that was carried out by our research group [13]. It deserves to be mentioned that oral chronic administration of PHT induces microsomal EPHX, which could explain why the percentage of subjects with toxicity is higher at the early stage of the treatment (healthy volunteers) than after a chronic one (patients participating in the pharmacovigilance program). A lesser exposure of reactive metabolite during chronic administration could be due to enzyme induction by PHT.

Although the number of ADRs was greater under Comitoína® treatment, the severity of such reactions was less intense as no seizures due to high concentrations was carried out reported.

One limitation of the study was self-reported data of ADRs when patients filled the form. This can inherently bias the number and severity of the reported reactions.

For both brands, when seizures and low concentrations were present, lack of efficacy was suspected, and then, the dose was immediately increased in order to achieve therapeutic concentrations.

Mean dose and mean plasma and salivary concentration of PHT that were able to control the seizures for Antepil® and Comitoína are shown in **Tables 6** and **7,** respectively.

As the three main enzymes that participate in PHT metabolism are polymorphically expressed and the genetic variants are responsible for changes in the enzyme activity, our research group has also evaluated the effect that these polymorphisms have on PHT metabolism. The genotypic frequencies obtained for CYPs are in accordance with the ones reported for Caucasian population [34]. Thirty percentage of the patients were intermediate, and 2% were poor metabolizers for CYP2C9, whereas 20% were intermediate metabolizers for CYP2C19. No poor metabolizer was found for CYP2C19. Regarding EPHX, 44% of the patients had an intermediate, 10% an increased, and 46% a decreased enzyme activity. Although 46% of the patients had a decreased EPHX activity, none of the patients reported cutaneous reactions. As it was stated, not only the detoxification pathway but also the rate of formation of this toxic metabolite (arene oxide) must be taken into account. Both formulations behave as slow-release tablets. Moreover, during chronic administration, a lesser exposure of reactive metabolite can be experienced due to the enzyme induction PHT provokes. Our results also evidenced a predominant role of CYP2C9 in PHT biotransformation, while CYP2C19 seems to have a predominant role in p-HPPH biotransformation [31].

Dose (mg/kg)	[Po] (mg/L)	[So] (mg/L)
4.03 (3.77–4.29)	7.12 (5.81–8.44)	0.626 (0.491–0.760)

Table 6.
Mean (95% CI) PHT dose and mean plasma and salivary concentrations in patients with controlled seizures under Antepil® treatment.

Dose (mg/kg)	[Po] (mg/L)	[So] (mg/L)
4.34 (4.12–4.55)	9.14 (8.08–10.2)	0.930 (0.780–1.08)

Table 7.
Mean (95% CI) PHT dose and mean plasma and salivary concentrations in patients with controlled seizures under Comitoína® treatment.

A bioequivalence parallel design study in saliva was also carried out with these data. According to the results obtained in this study, for the three parameters under evaluation (Css, Cmax, and PTF), bioequivalence between Antepil® and Comitoína® can be concluded. This procedure of parallel assay, with replicate evaluation of drug exposure, becomes a valuable solution to demonstrate bioequivalence of such products [35].

5. Conclusions

Both oral formulation of PHT show a uniform behavior in the population studied. The dose increase caused a disproportionate increase in plasma concentrations (Michaelis-Menten kinetics), as referenced in the literature.

No statistically significant differences were detected between the normalized doses received by both sexes or in the salivary concentrations or plasma concentrations obtained with such doses.

The presence of secondary peaks in salivary curves revealed the recirculation processes already known for PHT.

Adverse drug reactions referenced by patients did not deserve medical intervention in most cases, except for the appearance of seizures with high PHT concentrations.

CYP2C9 polymorphisms affect mainly PHT concentrations, while CYP2C19 polymorphisms affect mainly p-HPPH concentrations, which verify the predominant role that CYP2C9 has in PHT metabolism and CYP2C19 in p-HPPH metabolism. A decreased EPHX activity did not evidence arene oxide accumulation as no cutaneous reactions were observed.

According to the results obtained in the parallel study, switchability between the two commercial brands can be inferred.

In summary, mean (95% CI) PHT dose of 4.34 (4.12–4.55) mg/kg of Comitoína® and 4.03 (3.77–4.29) mg/kg of Antepil® achieved effective and safe concentrations of PHT.

Conflict of interest

The authors declare no conflict of interest.

Author details

Marta Vázquez[1*], Pietro Fagiolino[1], Cecilia Maldonado[1], Natalia Guevara[1],
Manuel Ibarra[1], Isabel Rega[2], Adriana Gómez[3], Antonella Carozzi[4]
and Carlos Azambuja[4]

1 Pharmaceutical Sciences Department, Faculty of Chemistry, Universidad de la
República, Montevideo, Uruguay

2 Neurology Clinics, Hospital Maciel, Montevideo, Uruguay

3 COSEM Clinics, Montevideo, Uruguay

4 Genia-Genetics Molecular Laboratory, Montevideo, Uruguay

*Address all correspondence to: mvazquez@fq.edu.uy

IntechOpen

References

[1] Goldenberg MM. Overview of drugs used for epilepsy and seizures. Etiology, diagnosis, and treatment. Pharmacy and Therapeutics. 2010;**35**(7):392-415

[2] Yaari Y, Selzer ME, Pincus JH. Phenytoin: Mechanisms of its anticonvulsant action. Annals of Neurology. 1986;**20**(2):171-184

[3] Patsalos PN, Berry DJ, Bourgeois BF, Cloyd JC, Glauser TA, Johannessen SI, et al. Antiepileptic drugs—Best practice guidelines for therapeutic drug monitoring: A position paper by the subcommission on therapeutic drug monitoring, ILAE Commission on Therapeutic Strategies. Epilepsia. 2008;**49**(7):1239-1276

[4] Maldonado C, Fagiolino P, Vázquez M, et al. Therapeutic carbamazepine (CBZ) and valproic acid (VPA) monitoring in children using saliva as a biologic fluid. Journal of Epilepsy and Clinical Neurophysiology. 2008;**14**(2):55-58

[5] Ibarra M, Vázquez M, Fagiolino P, Mutilva F, Canale A. Total, unbound plasma and salivary phenytoin levels in critically ill patients. Journal of Epilepsy and Clinical Neurophysiology. 2010;**16**(2):69-73

[6] Fagiolino P, Vázquez M, Maldonado C, et al. Usefulness of salivary drug monitoring for detecting efflux transporter overexpression. Current Pharmaceutical Design. 2013;**19**(38):6767-6774

[7] Posti J. Saliva-plasma drug concentration ratios during absorption: Theoretical considerations and pharmacokinetic implications. Pharmaceutica Acta Helvetiae. 1982;**57**:83-92

[8] Vázquez M, Fagiolino P, De Nucci G, Parrillo S, Piñeyro A. Post-prandial reabsorption of paracetamol. European Journal of Drug Metabolism and Pharmacokinetics. 1993 (Special Issue: 177-183. Proceedings of the 5th. Eur. Cong. Biopharm. Pharmacokinet., Brussel (Belgium), 1993)

[9] Vázquez M, Fagiolino P, Lorier M, Guevara N, Maldonado C, Ibarra M, Montes MJ, Retamoso I. Secondary-peak profile of methadone in saliva after administration of multiple doses in patients with chronic pain. Current Topics in Pharmacology. 2015;**19**:21-26

[10] Wu MF, Lim WH. Phenytoin: a guide to therapeutic drug monitoring. Proceedings of Singapore Healthcare. 2013;**22**:198-202

[11] Richens A. Clinical pharmacokinetics of phenytoin. Clinical Pharmacokinetics. 1979;**4**(3):153-169

[12] Thorn CF, Whirl-Carrillo M, Leeder JS, Klein TE, Altman RB. PharmGKB summary: Phenytoin pathway. Pharmacogenetics and Genomics. 2012;**22**:466-470

[13] Vázquez M, Fagiolino P, Alvariza S, Ibarra M, Maldonado C, Gonzalez R, Laborde A, Uria M, Carozzi A, Azambuja C. Skin reactions associated to phenytoin administration: Multifactorial cause. Clinical Pharmacology and Biopharmaceutics. 2014;**3**:125. doi: 10.4172/2167-065X.1000125

[14] Wormhoudt LW, Commandeur JN, Vermeulen NP. Genetic polymorphisms of human N-acetyltransferase, cytochrome P450, glutathione-S-transferase, and epoxide hydrolase enzymes: Relevance to xenobiotic metabolism and toxicity. Critical Reviews in Toxicology. 1999;**29**:59-124

[15] Ingelman-Sundberg M, Gaedigk A, Brockmöller J, Goldstein JA, Gonzalez

FJ, et al. The Human Cytochrome P450 (CYP) Allele Nomenclature Database. Available from: http://www.cypalleles. ki.se [Accessed: May 30, 2018]

[16] Pinarbasi H, Silig Y, Pinarbasi E. Microsomal epoxide hydrolase polymorphisms. Molecular Medicine Reports. 2010;**3**:723-727

[17] Mauro LS, Mauro VF, Brown DL, Somani P. Enhancement of phenytoin elimination by multiple-dose activated charcoal. Annals of Emergency Medicine. 1987;**16**:1132-1135

[18] Howard CE, Roberts RS, Ely DS, Moye RA. Use of multiple-dose activated charcoal in phenytoin toxicity. The Annals of Pharmacotherapy. 1994;**28**:201-203

[19] Glick TH, Workman TP, Graufberg SV. Preventing phenytoin intoxication: Safer use of a familiar anticonvulsant. The Journal of Family Practice. 2004;**53**:197-202

[20] Fagiolino P, Vázquez M, Eiraldi R, Maldonado C, Scaramelli A. Influence of efflux transporters on drug metabolism. Theoretical approach for bioavailability and clearance prediction. Clinical Pharmacokinetics. 2011;**50**:75-80

[21] Alvariza S, Fagiolino P, Vázquez M, Feria-Romero I, Orozco-Suárez S. Chronic administration of phenytoin induces efflux transporter overexpression in rats. Pharmacological Reports. 2014;**66**:946-951

[22] Alvariza S, Ibarra M, Vázquez M, Fagiolino P. Different phenytoin oral administration regimens could modify its chronic exposure and its saliva/plasma concentration ratio. Journal of Medical and Pharmaceutical Innovation. 2014;**1**:35-43

[23] Vázquez M, Fagiolino P, Mariño E. Concentration-dependent mechanisms of adverse drug reactions in epilepsy. Current Pharmaceutical Design. 2013;**19**:6802-6808

[24] Prasad K, Al-Roomi K, Krishnan PR, Sequeira R. Anticonvulsant therapy for status epilepticus. Cochrane Database of Systematic Reviews. 2005;**4**:CD003723. DOI: 10.1002/14651858.CD003723.pub2

[25] Browne TR, Kugler AR, Eldon MA. Pharmacology and pharmacokinetics of fosphenytoin. Neurology. 1996;**46**:S3-S7

[26] Jamerson BD, Dukes GE, Brouwer KL, Donn KH, Messenheimer JA, Powell JR. Venous irritation related to intravenous administration of phenytoin versus fosphenytoin. Pharmacotherapy. 1994;**14**:47-52

[27] Uribe-San-Martín R, Ciampi E, Uslar W, Villagra S, Plaza J, et al. Risk factors of early adverse drug reactions with phenytoin: A prospective inpatient cohort. Epilepsy & Behavior. 2017;**76**:139-144

[28] Brodie MJ, Mintzer S, Pack AM, Gidal BE, Vecht CJ, Schmidt D. Enzyme induction with antiepileptic drugs: Cause for concern? Epilepsia. 2013;**54**:11-27

[29] Chung WH, Wang CW, Dao RL. Severe cutaneous adverse drug reactions. The Journal of Dermatology. 2016;**43**:758-766

[30] Savio E, Fagiolino P, Solana G, Parente E, León A. Development of water/oil emulsion. Bioavailability in rats. STP Pharma Sciences. 1991;**1**:379-385

[31] Guevara N, Maldonado C, Uría M, González R, Ibarra M, et al. Role of CYP2C9, CYP2C19 and EPHX polymorphism in the pharmacokinetic of phenytoin: A study on Uruguayan Caucasian subjects. Pharmaceuticals. 2017;**10**:73. DOI: 10.3390/ ph10030073

[32] Vázquez M, Fagiolino P, Maldonado C, et al. Hyperammonemia associated with valproic acid concentrations. BioMed Research International. 2014;**2014**:217269. DOI: 10.1155/2014/217269

[33] Maldonado C, Guevara N, Queijo C, et al. Carnitine and/or acetylcarnitine deficiency as a cause of higher levels of ammonia. BioMed Research International. 2016;**2016**:2920108. DOI: 10.1155/2016/2920108

[34] Lee CR, Goldstein JA, Pieper JA. Cytochrome P450 2C9polymorphisms: A comprehensive review of the *in-vitro* and human data. Pharmacogenetics. 2002;**12**:251-263

[35] Guevara N, Fagiolino P, Vázquez M, Maldonado C. Replicate evaluation of drug exposure to study bioequivalence between two brands of phenytoin in patients. Current Topics in Pharmacology. 2018;**22** (in press)

9 781789 857597